Knowing how to recover from life's inevitable disappointments and emotional injuries is an essential skill for successful relationships. Worthington and Ripley offer a practical, sensitive, and evidence-based approach for helping couples to recover from relationship wounds and pursue a joyful life together. This marvelous new text provides step-by-step interventions for promoting hope and forgiveness and is an indispensable resource for every couple therapist.

Douglas K. Snyder, Ph.D., is Professor of Psychological and Brain Sciences at Texas A&M University (College Station). Co-author of *Getting Past the Affair*, Co-editor of the *Clinical Handbook of Couple Therapy*

Here is a book with a difference. The Hope-Focused Couples Approach (HFCA) is packed with more practical suggestions than one could hope for and it creates hope in both couples and therapists. It is technique-heavy and can be integrated with virtually any approach to couple therapy. You can select those techniques that fit into your treatment and add new methods of positive psychology are deigned to promote forgiveness, humility, gratitude, and hope. HFCA provides authoritative coverage of forgiveness and reconciliation for couples based on the authors' extensive research and practice on these processes. I believe you'll find this book a hands-on, practical resource.

Leslie Greenberg, Distinguished Research Professor Emeritus, Dept. of Psychology, York University, Toronto Ontario

After 30 years practicing couple therapy, I would describe it as a challenging but deeply rewarding adventure, and one that definitely requires a good "map." In this book, Worthington and Ripley have provided an outstanding *map* based on their Hope-Focused Couple Approach drawing on a textured theoretical framework, solid research evidence, and a flexible set of interventions for effectively engaging couples' strengths and values toward healing and growth. I grew to love doing couple therapy using an early version of this approach during my graduate training, and I continue to benefit from the clinical wisdom and strategic clarity of these authors as their model has evolved. I consider this book essential reading in the field of couple therapy.

Steven J. Sandage, Ph.D., LP, Boston University

This book offers an indispensable roadmap for forming, growing, maintaining, and repairing the emotional bond. Covering topics ranging from how to get couples to do homework, to understanding what to do when the emotional bond is severely strained, to immensely practical strategies to tackle such big and potentially overwhelming constructs like hope and forgiveness, this is a fantastic tool box for both new therapists and seasoned ones alike. I learned many new strategies that I look forward to implementing in my own practice. One of this book's greatest contributions to the literature is the concept of hope, which is an overlooked virtue in couple relationships. As long as couples have hope and commitment, they can surmount daily fluctuations in their satisfaction and retain motivation to work toward change. Loss of hope is deadly, and I am grateful that these two excellent therapists have brought this concept front and center of this book so that other therapists will pay attention to it and learn how to cultivate it when it is waning.

Kristina Coop Gordon, Ph.D. Professor and Associate Dean for Community Engagement University of Tennessee-Knoxville. Co-author of *Getting Past the Affair*

This book is the first to provide an innovative, practice friendly integration of constructs in positive psychology into couple therapy. The numerous interventions provided throughout the text are explained within a patient-friendly framework that will appeal to all therapists regardless of theoretical orientation. It is an essential resource that belongs on the shelves of novice to seasoned practitioners.

Frank D. Fincham, Ph.D. Eminent Scholar and Director, Florida State University Family Institute

This book, written by two true experts in couples' relationships, incorporates a rare combination of strategies to inspire hope, positivity, and forgiveness for couples in an easy-to-understand, practical manner. It is filled with empirically supported strategies that will be invaluable across therapists' theoretical orientations while providing a cogent, flexible framework for treatment. This volume will expand and deepen the work of both experienced and beginning couple therapists, and I recommend it highly.

Don Baucom Distinguished Professor of Psychology and Neuroscience University of North Carolina. Co-author of Baucom, D. H., Fischer, M. S., Corrie, S., Worrell, M., & Boeding, S. E., *Treating relationship distress and psychopathology in couples: A cognitive-behavioural approach* (2020)

Worthington and Ripley have expanded the boundaries of couple therapy, covering all the twists and turns from intake to termination, as well as providing a rich conceptual framework to guide intervention. Their detailed description of over 100 practical strategies to help couples as they strengthen their relationships and build hope for the future is a wonderful addition to the field and a must read for students, teachers, scholars, and practitioners in the ever-evolving field of couple therapy.

Steven R. H. Beach, Ph.D. Regent's Professor of Psychology, University of Georgia Director, Center for Family Research Author, Depression in Marriage

This is an exceptional resource for marital and couples therapists of any theoretical background. Centered around the goal of producing hope, Worthington and Ripley provide over 100 clear, usable—"how to do it"—strategies. The work is richly cited, engaging, and thoroughly useful.

Scott M. Stanley, Ph.D. Research Professor, University of Denver. Co-author of *Fighting for Your Marriage*

Hope, Forgiveness, and Positive Psychology in Couple Therapy

This guide introduces the Hope-Focused Approach to couple therapy and provides a hands-on, practical resource for clinicians and students to integrate this approach into their practice effectively.

Drawing from positive psychology, virtue theory, and forgiveness theory, the book describes how therapists can design a hope-focused treatment to promote intimacy, help couples communicate and resolve disagreements, strengthen emotional bonds, build trust, guide forgiveness, and encourage reconciliation. This book takes the therapist from assessing couples, to designing initial treatment plans, intervening in sessions, and facilitating termination. Focusing on communication training and conflict resolution, Worthington and Ripley share over 100 evidence-based techniques, case studies, and interventions to illustrate how to help couples effectively. Examples incorporate complex issues of race and sexuality, as well as values such as religion and politics. This practical guide arms therapists with a strategy to enrich their practice of couple therapy, equips them with practical techniques, and helps them promote forgiveness and reconciliation when couples seek it.

This book is an invaluable resource for beginning counselors, graduate students, and practicing marriage and family therapists.

Everett L. Worthington Jr. is a clinical psychologist and Commonwealth Professor Emeritus at Virginia Commonwealth University. He has had over 40 years of licensed practice and has written almost 50 books on topics such as forgiveness, couple therapy, and spirituality/religion.

Jennifer S. Ripley is a professor of Clinical Psychology at Regent University, Virginia, sharing the Hughes Chair for Integration of Mental Health. As a licensed clinical psychologist, she directs the couple lab at Regent University, supervises many couple therapists, and sees dozens of couples per year, testing the ideas for this book in a real-world therapeutic setting. Her website is www.hopecouples.com.

Hope, Forgiveness, and Positive Psychology in Couple Therapy

Everett L. Worthington Jr. and
Jennifer S. Ripley

Routledge
Taylor & Francis Group
NEW YORK AND LONDON

Designed cover image: © Getty images

First published 2025
by Routledge
605 Third Avenue, New York, NY 10158

and by Routledge
4 Park Square, Milton Park, Abingdon, Oxon, OX14 4RN

Routledge is an imprint of the Taylor & Francis Group, an informa business

Library of Congress Cataloging-in-Publication Data
Names: Worthington, Everett L., Jr., 1946– author. |
Ripley, Jennifer S., 1972– author.
Title: Hope, forgiveness, and positive psychology in couple therapy /
Everett L. Worthington Jr. and Jennifer S. Ripley.
Description: New York, NY : Routledge, 2025. |
Includes bibliographical references and index.
Identifiers: LCCN 2024029522 (print) | LCCN 2024029523 (ebook) |
ISBN 9780367443825 (hardback) | ISBN 9780367443849
(paperback) | ISBN 9781003009382 (ebook)
Subjects: MESH: Couples Therapy | Hope | Forgiveness |
Psychology, Positive
Classification: LCC RC488.5 .W678 2025 (print) | LCC RC488.5
(ebook) | NLM WM 430.5.M3 | DDC 616.89/1562—dc23/eng/
20240702
LC record available at https://lccn.loc.gov/2024029522
LC ebook record available at https://lccn.loc.gov/2024029523

ISBN: 978-0-367-44382-5 (hbk)
ISBN: 978-0-367-44384-9 (pbk)
ISBN: 978-1-003-00938-2 (ebk)

DOI: 10.4324/9781003009382

Typeset in Sabon LT Pro
by Apex CoVantage, LLC

To Don Danser, the first Christian doctoral student I had the pleasure of advising. Don is a wonderful man of God. The couple that got me started looking at forgiveness intervention was Don and his wife, and we developed in collaboration a brief intervention to help them consider forgiveness. Don, a psychotherapist for many years, has always been willing to serve and has always been an inspiration to me.

—Ev

To Bob and Genelda Sulouff, from whose beautiful marriage I owe my very fortunate life.

—Jen

Contents

Acknowledgments

We are grateful to Pastor Doug McMurry, who was, at one time, pastor to both of us at Christ Presbyterian Church in Richmond, Virginia, and his lifetime wife and companion, Carla. But after Doug left CPC, he and Carla established a retreat center. Ev's wife of 53 years, Kirby, had had numerous serious medical complications, which was resulting in a serious approach-to-deadline without even starting to draft this book. But Doug made a way by allowing Ev to take a writing retreat at the McMurrys, which allowed almost all of the book's first draft to be written. This book would not have come about without the McMurrys' generosity.

Jen's favorite artist, and youngest child, L. Ripley created the artwork for the book. Dropping out of college to redirect your life never produced better stuff! I'm deeply grateful you offered your talents to this endeavor.

We are very thankful to Gabriella Jones for her work in assisting with references throughout the book and for her unending joyful spirit.

Jen also acknowledges with gratitude the many former graduate students who have contributed ideas, conducted research, and pilot tested so many of the ideas of this book. In particular, I am grateful to those who have led the research management or conducted dissertations in Hope-Focused Couple Therapy (HFCT): Rhonda Ladd, Anna Ord, Cynthia Leon, Anastasia Whitesell, Candance Lassiter, Caroline Bridges, Elizabeth Wine, Raquel Hatcher, Stacey Villanueva, Aleksandra Wantke, Lindsay Solfelt, Nicole Urh, Amy Robertson, Camden Pigg, Amber Perkins, Tiffany Channing, Vera Turbessi, Genevieve Maksad, Gabby Jones, and Faith Malone.

We are also so appreciative of the effort put into conducting research on the HFCT to establish its long-term effectiveness and its use in actual couple therapy. This involves funders (like Scott Richards and the John Templeton Foundation), many co-authors (e.g., Job Chen, Vanessa Kent, and Elizabeth Loewer, just to mention some recent ones), numerous research assistants, and countless couple therapists and their brave couples who trusted those therapists. Thank you all!

We gratefully acknowledge the wonderful team at Routledge that we were privileged to work with on this book. They have been always helpful and very patient with us. This included Clare Ashworth, with whom we worked in the early development, and Ellie Duncan, her assistant. But in its full development, we have really appreciated the encouragement and feedback by Julia Giordano and the final preparation work of Gillian Steadman.

Preface

You can enrich your practice of couple therapy by learning over 100 new intervention methods, most of which will fit with the couple therapy you now use. We use the hope-focused couple approach (HFCA) as a springboard. If you have not adopted the HFCA already, we believe you will still become a more effective couple therapist by working through this book.

This Approach and These Methods Can Fit with Your Approach

The HFCA is methodologically *pluralistic* (see Lebow & Snyder, 2022). While starting as a strategic theory in the late 1970s, over the years, the HFCA has incorporated methods and techniques of couple therapy seamlessly from many theories:

- Family systems therapies: problem-solving therapy, structural family therapy, solution-focused therapy, Bowenian therapy, and narrative therapy
- Behavioral couple therapies: integrative behavioral couple therapy, cognitive-behavioral couple therapy, and Acceptance and Commitment Therapy
- Emotion-centered couple therapies: emotion-focused couple therapy, Gottman couple therapy
- Spiritually integrated couple therapy: Worthington's Christian couple counseling and the spiritually integrated therapies developed by P. Scott Richards and Ken Pargament, among others.

Approaches that are pluralistic (sometimes called integrative) are not eclectic (Lebow & Snyder, 2023). Technical eclecticism was originally championed by Arnold Lazarus, who argued that techniques could be used from any therapy if they met one criterion: they worked. Eclecticism has been criticized because methods from different approaches may work at cross-purposes to each other. For example, psychodynamic approaches tend to uncover conflicts and resistances and then interpret the dynamics within them. Cognitive and behavioral approaches tend to be based on cooperation. Using techniques from both risks confusing clients as to whether they should cooperate with or resist the therapist. Of course, it is possible to put the two together (see Wachtel, 2014). But this requires an overarching theoretical perspective that the clients are helped to understand. The other major danger of eclecticism is that the therapist might pull a technique that won't work on its own from a complex approach that works as a whole. Removing the technique from its usual context might gut its effectiveness.

The HFCA is methodologically pluralistic. We trust that you can read the techniques we recommend and select those that fit into your treatment. We trust that you won't select those that are inherently incompatible with your overall approach. We believe that most of the techniques we recommend have been tested and found to work as we present them. Thus, if you do not adapt further, these methods should work in your practice.

Evidence-Based Couple Therapy

The HFCA has sought to be evidence-based from its outset. We have published lab-based randomized controlled efficacy trials (Worthington et al., 1997) and community-based effectiveness trials (Ripley et al., 2014, 2023). We have studied important aspects of the HFCA split in half. In Worthington et al. (2015), we compared HOPE (handling our problems effectively), which includes formal assessment plus treatment of communication problems, conflict resolution, and intimacy promotion, against FREE (forgiveness and reconciliation through experiencing empathy). Each was effective but had different effects. In Worthington et al. (1989), we examined other aspects of couple treatment, including brief modules on communication, conflict, and intimacy (each made a contribution) and the effects of group treatments versus individual meetings with a facilitator (individual was better). In Worthington et al. (1995), we compared the effects of assessment and feedback sessions against assessment only (getting the full assessment with feedback helped enormously). We have done extensive research on both forgiveness and reconciliation. Over 30 randomized controlled trials have been done worldwide on the REACH forgiveness method (Worthington, 2006), showing it very effective.

Most of the studies have been on a secular version of the HFCA. But a few have studied the use of a spiritually accommodated approach (Hook et al., 2014; Ripley et al., 2022). Some have even compared the secular with a Christian-accommodated approach, finding no difference in relational outcomes with Christian couples (Ripley et al., 2014). We have found good effect sizes in following up with couple-therapy clients for up to ten years post-therapy (Ripley et al., 2023).

We are confident the method as a whole, in part, and the techniques will work for your clients. And speaking of techniques, positive psychology of forgiveness, humility, gratitude, and hope provide meaning and substance to HFCA, and also contribute proven-effective techniques.

- Positive psychology studies forgiveness. We describe many techniques to help you use forgiveness interventions. These include seeking, experiencing, communicating, and accepting forgiveness. Also, forgiveness can be a launching platform for reconciliation, self-forgiveness, and even (sometimes) experiencing forgiveness by God.
- Positive psychology studies humility. In research, we have found that a lack of humility in couples can quickly sour interactions. So, we describe how you can encourage it.
- Positive psychology studies gratitude. Feeling gratitude for the partner and expressing it can re-orient relationships (see Davis et al., 2016).
- Positive psychology studies hope. Hope is obviously a key to our approach to couple therapy. We endorse and build on the cognitive model of hope as agency and pathways thinking that C. R. Snyder (1994) introduced in the 1990s. We incorporate persevering hope, which is crucial to couples who enter couple therapy believing that their relationship is doomed (Rueger et al., 2022. For some, eschatological hope (i.e., a theological term meaning ultimate hope in God; Witvliet et al., 2022) can be an aid to their relationship restoration.

Not surprisingly, if you've been a couple therapist for a while, you'll recognize that your own hope can play a role in successful therapy. Who hasn't found that we, at times, need hope to persevere when couples have a terrible session or tumultuous week between sessions.

Congratulations! If you are not a big fan of reading research summaries, you have now weathered the most research-intensive section of the book. Yes, there will be other mentions of research, but we wanted to give you enough summary and references that, if you are interested, you can follow up. Also, we want you to know that what we are saying is informed *both* by practice and research.

The HFCA Has a Consistent Unifying Theory

The HFCA has a coherent theory uniting it. It is focused on hope, strategically driven, and technique-heavy. We are not trying to convert you to the

HFCA theory, even though we will briefly explain the theory so you see its coherence. Rather, we are taking advantage of the technical pluralism of the method to provide practical techniques that will fit into *your* approach to couple therapy to enrich your practice.

How You Can Use This Book

You can use this book (and approach) in four ways. First, the HFCA can stand on its own as an evidence-based treatment, if you wish to use it intact. Second, the HFCA can be integrated with virtually any approach to couple therapy, to provide a coherent meta-theory and to organize the practical, therapy-tested (and often research-proven) techniques of couple therapy. Third, even if you don't adopt the approach whole-cloth, you can extract your favorites from over 100 practical, couple-therapy tested methods. Those can enrich your repertoire of interventions. Fourth, among all of the couple approaches, the HFCA provides the most authoritative coverage of forgiveness and reconciliation for couples based on Worthington's extensive research and practice with forgiveness and reconciliation. We believe clinicians and clinicians-in-training will find this book to be a hands-on, practical resource.

In 2015, Gurman, Lebow, and Snyder brought out the fifth edition of the authoritative *Clinical Handbook of Couple Therapy* shortly after Alan Gurman's passing. Now, in 2023, they have produced the most recent *Handbook* (Lebow & Snyder, 2023; sixth edition). It demonstrates how the theoretical pantheon of couple therapy approaches used today were largely developed between 1980 and 2000. Most of the approaches are focused on a single theory. Behaviorally oriented and cognitively oriented approaches appeal to the behaviorally inclined. The emotionally focused approach appeals to those who see emotion as primary in relationships. The psychoanalytically informed approach appeals to those who already are psychoanalytically inclined or who look to partners' past for clues about their relationship. Lebow and Snyder grouped them with other multigenerational approaches. Post-structural and social constructionist approaches appeal to those who engage with a philosophy that emphasizes the influence of identity and diversity on relationships. Finally, some approaches are frankly integrative. They employ many techniques and methods from different approaches, yet they have an overarching narrative that ties together the methods. Lebow and Snyder (2023) include common factors (Davis, 2023), integrative systemic therapy for couples (Breunlin et al., 2023), therapeutic palette integrative couple therapy (Fraenkel, 2023), and the Gottman method couple therapy (Gottman & Gottman, 2023). Traditional systemic approaches, such as structural and strategic approaches which appealed to systems theorists in earlier decades, may still have historical influence but have largely been abandoned except by clinicians who have long practiced them. A glimmer of those old family systems theories shines from integrative systemic therapy (see Breunlin et al., 2023).

If Lebow and Snyder (2023) had included HFCA in their classification system, we probably would find it among the integrative approaches. In our thinking, however, we would not place this book in that camp. We are not trying to be dismissive of the new or old pantheon of theories. But to us, it seems that most practicing couple therapists are not theoretically identified. One might think most therapists would identify with one of the integrative approaches. But it seems that most practitioners today either describe themselves as drawing techniques eclectically, or they might identify with a specific approach, but at least sometimes use other approaches. Those practical therapists, who are willing to use what works, are the ones this book is for. Regardless of what theoretical approach you identify with, we believe that you can find new methods—and we hope new thoughts—to enrich your practice.

Our Roots: Our Debt to Other Practitioners

We owe a great debt to many couple therapies, and the theorists and practitioners who have developed them. We start with those because we believe human relationships are at least as important as the abstracted theories that come from personal experiences—with clients, research findings, and their personal life experiences of the theorists. We've seen some great couple therapists in action over the years. While you might not recognize many of these people, we are sure you have similar therapists who have influenced you, and perhaps this will help you reflect on them.

We begin to honor our debt by mentioning how we have greatly influenced each other as psychologists, counselors, and friends for many years. At the beginning of her career, Jen was a student who worked with Ev, but that was always more of a collaboration to help couples than a traditional student–teacher relationship. So, we will just take for granted that you know that we have shaped each other's thinking about treating couples.

For Ev, perhaps one of the most influential therapists was Carl Rilee. Carl was a social worker in Richmond, about 15 years older than Ev. When Ev first came to Richmond in 1978, to take up a position at Virginia Commonwealth University, he met Carl at a meeting of family practitioners. Somehow, they clicked. Carl became Ev's unofficial supervisor while Ev was receiving licensure supervision from Donald Kiesler and Stanley Strong—both for couple therapy—and Robert Tipton for individual therapy.

Carl was a gentle, soft-spoken man who invited Ev and Kirby over to his and his wife's home. They formed a couple-based friendship. "Carl would come down to the VCU area about monthly," says Ev, "and we would have a soda at the Burger King [BK] behind my building. Lots of informal supervision went on at BK. What he taught me was the importance of warmth and connection—not just as a therapist but as a human. Although Carl had been in general practice for probably 25 years, he actually asked my advice on some cases. I also shared my struggles as a budding therapist and learned from his experience. I saw him counsel. He was a master. I wish I had had the wisdom to systematically observe him to figure out what he did to make such an impact on his clients. I probably referred 50 couples to him over the years. And as the highest testimony, I received only praise for Carl from the people I referred."

Don Kiesler was one of Carl Rogers' colleagues in his days at the University of Wisconsin. Rogers was one of the founders of person-centered psychology. Don wrote one of the 12 featured articles by the American Psychological Association in celebrating the first 100 years of psychology—on the interpersonal circle. Don had joined the faculty as a senior clinical psychologist about two years before Ev joined the faculty as the rookie counseling psychologist. Don gave Ev perhaps his most memorable moment in supervision. He describes it this way. "Don listened attentively to my description of a case about which I had almost given up hope. He was a world-class listener! When my energy ran down, Don just sat there for about 15 seconds. Then he pushed forward until he was sitting on the edge of his chair and said, 'Okay. Here's what we're going to do!' At that moment, I thought I could fly. Hope rushed in with eagle wings."

Both of these formative supervisor–influencers emphasized the power of the interpersonal relationship of supervisor on supervisee, of clinician on patient, and of friends being human with each other. Somehow that stuck. "I tried to be as warm and therapeutic as Carl Rogers, who was one of my heroes," says Ev. "One of the graduate students in our doctoral program at one time mused about my influence on her counseling style. 'You remind me of someone really famous,' she said. I immediately puffed up, thinking of Sean Connery. 'Yes,' she said, 'it's Rogers.' Okay, well. That immediately dashed my roguishly good-looks fantasy. But still. Carl Rogers was not too bad. I don't think I actually said, 'Aw, shucks' and scuffed my toe modestly. But, I admit I was thinking about it. Then she said, 'Yeah. You remind me of *Mr.* Rogers.' Oh. Fred."

"Okay, on occasion, I can be flexible. The next day, I came into the practicum class, walking slowly and deliberately. I took off my blazer. Pulled a cardigan off the hook behind the door, changed in slow motion into my tennis shoes, and got down to serious teaching about psychotherapy—not into NOM (the Neighborhood of Make-Believe)."

Ev's third most influential couple therapist was Steve Sandage. Steve was a student in the doctoral program and a few years earlier than Jen.

Steve was, from the beginning, a mature and wise psychotherapist and human. "I never saw a situation in which he wasn't in control," said Ev. He has always been a big fan of Bowen's concept of ego differentiation. That fit Steve. He was able to value people regardless of the emotion swirling around him. He refused to be fused to toxic emotion, but he was warm, connected emotionally, attuned, and a wise problem-solver—an exemplar of "differentiation of self."

Ev reflected on his mentors. Perhaps this might have stimulated you to also do so. "Looking back," he says, "I see that the people who most influenced me as a therapist also influenced me as a person. They were students (Jen and Steve), teacher (Don), and friend (Carl). But each was my teacher in therapy and in life."

For Jen, "My largest influence in couple therapy training is my professor and friend Ev Worthington, who took on this 22-year-old naïve graduate student in 1994. When we met, it was a mind-meld, like meeting a much smarter and more experienced brain that seemed to know my own thoughts before I could form them. For more reflections on his unique brand of Mr. Roger's kindness and Sean Connery wit, clearly displayed in the story of showing up to class dressed as Mr. Rogers, see Ripley (2024). Ev invited me into his home too (as Rilee had done with Ev) where I met and became friends with his wife Kirby, a woman who has been very important to me. His couple therapy class set the standard for learning the practical work of couple therapy. He proved I could trust him in this work, to actually help couples in ways that appeared simple and accessible, even to the most emotionally-flooded partner with limited resources, but were actually quite sophisticated in science and theory."

Steve Sandage's ideas on differentiation and diversity have also influenced Jen's clinical work. "Steve's been an academic big brother for decades," Jen observes. "I feel we must give some credit to the Christ Presbyterian community in Richmond as well, where we all, Ev, Steve, and I learned and grew together in ways that are hard to fully appreciate from such a short time together."

Jen says that the Hope lab at Regent University has been a joy to learn deeply from dozens of graduate students who spend four years seeing cases and working tirelessly for the good of couples. She says that forming this training lab in 2007 was her best professional decision. It allowed her to learn from the couples and students what works with both couples and therapists-in-training and what they each need. The graduate students creatively contributed to the ideas, and perhaps most importantly kept Jen's feet to the ground, continually seeking out what *actually works* with the many struggling couples who found our lab. Over 500 couples have come through that lab in some way, and they deserve credit for their investment in their ideas. "I must say," says Jen, "the weekly Hope supervision group with 4th-year doctoral students is always my favorite hour of the week."

"I also have strong influences from emotion-focused couple therapy and family system theory. One former grad student from 2008 transformed to become my closest friend, Dr. Rhonda Ladd, an excellent EFCT counselor who keeps emotions on my mind while walking Saturday mornings in our favorite park.

"For the last five years, Jim Sells has been a voluntary co-supervisor of the Hope project and brother to me as we co-direct the Charis Institute. He lives well as a family man in life, and an excellent family therapist. My increasing ability to be a non-anxious presence and differentiated is because I have pinged off Jim's family systems-soaked visionary brain. Many of my recent Hope-focused ideas originate in conversations with Rhonda and Jim."

We debated whether to include this last section on people who influenced us. In the end, though, we saw it as crucial. Being an excellent individual, couple, or family therapist is not merely a matter of learning 100 new counseling techniques or having a coherent meta-theory to guide counseling. In the end, it's about human-to-human relationships. Couples are struggling, and we are just frail humans seeking to enter their struggles and stand with them until they—at least we hope—emerge at peace.

References

Breunlin, D. C., Russell, W. P., Chambers, A. L., & Solomon, A. R. (2023). Integrative systemic therapy for couples. In J. L. Lebow & D. K. Snyder (Eds.), *Clinical Handbook of Couple Therapy,* 6th *ed.* (pp. 318–338). The Guilford Press.

Davis, D. E., Choe, E., Meyers, J., Wade, N. G., Varjas, K., Gifford, A., Quinn, A., Hook, J. N., Van Tongeren, D. R., Griffin, B. J., Worthington, E. L., Jr. (2016). Thankful for the little things: A meta-analysis of gratitude interventions. *Journal of Counseling Psychology, 63*(1), 20–31.

Davis, S. (2023). Common factors in couple therapy. In J. L. Lebow & D. K. Snyder (Eds.), *Clinical Handbook of Couple Therapy,* 6th *ed.* (pp. 295–317). The Guilford Press.

Fraenkel, P. (2023). Therapeutic palette integrative couple therapy. In J. L. Lebow & D. K. Snyder (Eds.), *Clinical Handbook of Couple Therapy,* 6th *ed.* (pp. 339–361). The Guilford Press.

Gottman, J. M., & Gottman, J. S. (2023). The Gottman method couple therapy. In J. L. Lebow & D. K. Snyder (Eds.), *Clinical Handbook of Couple Therapy,* 6th *ed.* (pp. 362–386). The Guilford Press.

Gurman, A. S., Lebow, J. L., & Snyder, D. K. (Eds.). (2015). *Clinical Handbook of Couple Therapy,* 5th *ed.* The Guilford Press.

Hook, J. N., Worthington, E. L., Jr., Atkins, D., & Davis, D. E. (2014). Religion and couple therapy: Description and preliminary outcome data. *Psychology of Religion and Spirituality,* 6(2), 94–101.

Lebow, J. L., & Snyder, D. K. (2022). Couple therapy in the 2020s: Current status and emerging developments. *Family Process, 61,* 1359–1385. https://doi.org/10.1111/faam.12824

Lebow, J. L., & Snyder, D. K. (Eds.). (2023). *Clinical Handbook of Couple Therapy,* 6th *ed*. The Guilford Press.

Ripley, J. S. (2024). Everett Worthington: Lessons in over 25 years and counting. *Spirituality in Clinical Practice Special Issue*. In press.

Ripley, J. S., Leon, C., Worthington, E. J., Berry, J. W., Davis, E. B., Smith, A., Atkinson, A., & Sierra, T. (2014). Efficacy of religion-accommodative strategic hope-focused theory applied to couples therapy. *Couple and Family Psychology: Research and Practice, 3*, 83–98.

Ripley, J., Solfelt, L., Ord, A., Garthe, R. C., Worthington, E. L., Jr., & Channing, T. (2023). Short- and long-term outcomes of hope focused couple therapy. *Spirituality in Clinical Practice, 10*(4), 271–288. https://doi.org/10.1037/scp0000286 publication. https://doi.org/10.1037/scp0000286

Ripley, J. S., Worthington, E. L., Jr., Kent, V., Loewer, E., & Chen, Z. J. (2022). Community-based spiritually integrated couple therapy: Christian-accommodated couple therapy as an illustration. *Psychotherapy*, *59*(3), 382–391.

Rueger, S. Y., Worthington, Jr., E. L., Davis, E. B., Chen, Z. J., Cowden, R. G., Moloney, J. M., . . . Glowiak, K. J. (2022). Development and initial validation of the persevering hope scale: Measuring wait-power in four independent samples. *Journal of Personality Assessment*, *105*(1), 58–73. https://doi.org/10.1080/00223891.2022.2032100

Snyder, C. R. (1994). *The Psychology of Hope*. The Free Press.

Wachtel, P. L. (2014). An integrative relational point of view. *Psychotherapy, 51,* 342–349.

Witvliet, C. V. O., Hall, M. E. L., Exline, J., Wang, D. C., Root Luna, L M., Van Tongeren, D. R., Myers, D. G., Abernethy, A. D., & Witvliet, J. D. (2022). The Eschatological Hope Scale: Construct development and measurement of theistic eschatological hope. *Journal of Psychology and Christianity*, *41*(1), 16–35.

Worthington, E. L., Jr. (2006). *Forgiveness and Reconciliation: Theory and Application*. Brunner-Routledge.

Worthington, E. L., Jr., Berry, J. W., Hook, J. N., Davis, D. E., Scherer, M., Griffin, B. J., Wade, N. G., Yarhouse, M., Ripley, J. S., Miller, A. J., Sharp, C. B, Canter, D. E., & Campana, K. L. (2015). Forgiveness-reconciliation and communication-conflict-resolution interventions versus rested controls in early married couples. *Journal of Counseling Psychology*, *62*(1), 14–27.

Worthington, E. L., Jr., Buston, B. G., & Hammonds, T. M. (1989). A component analysis of marriage enrichment: Information and treatment modality. *Journal for Counseling and Development, 67, 555–560.*

Worthington, E. L., Jr., Hight, T. L., Ripley, J. S., Perrone, K. M., Kurusu, T. A., & Jones, D. R. (1997). Strategic hope-focused relationship-enrichment counseling with individual couples. *Journal of Counseling Psychology, 44*, 381–389.

Worthington, E. L., Jr., McCullough, M. E., Shortz, J. L., Mindes, E. J., Sandage, S. J., & Chartrand, J. M. (1995). Can marital assessment and feedback improve marriages? Assessment as a brief marital enrichment procedure. *Journal of Counseling Psychology, 42, 466–475.*

1 Admitting to the Fragility of Couple Therapy

Hold On To Hope

It works for the Marvel Universe: Begin with the origin story. So, we thought we'd try it.

Ev's Origin Story

I (Ev) remember my licensure case. This was back in the days when we had to walk to the office, in the snow, uphill, both ways. Okay, it was only 1981. For licensure, we not only had to pass the national psychologist exam, but also a thorough state exam on ethics and law in Virginia, submit a work sample showing how we assess and treat clients from the population we hoped to work with, and then undergo a Torquemada-inspired oral exam. After almost three post-PhD years of seeing clients under supervision, I created my 50-single-spaced-page (no pictures) work sample. I presented a brief couple-therapy case with six sessions. Of course, the couple had not completed their last session, but a successful termination session was planned for the afternoon, and we all know that those are successful 100 percent of the time. After that session, I would write a (humble but) glowing report of the termination and hand-deliver the case study to the Board of Psychology by the deadline. And then wait for the accolades to roll in.

The partners settled in. "How was your week?" Always good to have a snappy opening for a celebratory session.

"Uh, not too good," said the husband, whom I'll call Jared.

"Really?" My voice didn't really crack, although it elevated an octave. "What happened?"

They unfolded a scenario from hell—at least as far as my plans for licensure were concerned. It began with a visit by Jared's parents and a benevolent offer to take their family—Jared, his one-year-old son Jon, and wife Allison—to Virginia Beach for the day. But Allison didn't want to go. As the mother, she claimed that Jon was staying home with her. An argument

DOI: 10.4324/9781003009382-1

ensued. Allison expected Jared to side with her. Jared sided with his parents. So, Allison scooped up Jon and ran to the car, locking herself inside. Jared and his parents pursued.

"These big huge adults surrounded my car, shouting at us. They tried to take my baby!" she wailed. She refused to come out until the in-laws left.

"Now," she said. "We want a divorce." Jared nodded.

Inside my head, explosions went off. My noise-shy career as a therapist took flight. I didn't think the Board of Psychology would be impressed with this turn of events. There was stunned silence in the room. I held up my hand in a "Wait" gesture. "I need a little time." I was actually videotaping that session because I was still under supervision, as was the policy of our clinic. I also had the couple's permission to tape because I was using the case for licensure. So, I put my head down. I hid my eyes. Not ideal license-competent therapist behavior. About one and a half minutes of silence ensured. I contemplated what to do. (Not really. Instead, I just listened to the screaming voice in my head yelling, "You're a failure!") It seemed like hours.

I'd like to say that I came up with some brilliant intervention to turn the session into a complete success. I didn't. But a glimmer of hope entered my psychological darkness. I started by observing that they were having a power struggle over their child. (My insight is legendary.) I asked whether they could solve this themselves. They couldn't.

So, I offered to flip a coin and let chance resolve whether the child would stay with the husband or wife. That was, as they say, wildly rejected (as I had hoped it would be). So, I asked them what was important to them. As they talked, the uncomfortable truth came to them. They did not want solutions. They did not want a win–win. They each wanted to WIN. I suggested that placing their child in the center, one might eventually win, but it likely would tear the child apart. Both professed too much love for the child to continue their blood sport. I said that there were ways that win–win solutions could emerge if they hung in there. They agreed to keep coming back.

I showed that videotape repeatedly in training graduate students and in teaching couple therapy. That was not my finest therapeutic moment. But, I at least talked them off of the ledge and got them back the next week, and the next, and the next. Turns out they were far from termination.

The Board of Psychology was understanding. I'm sure this was not the only couple that blew up in the history of Virginia Clinical Psychology. And I did get my license.

But the next few weeks were a period of deep hopelessness for me. I questioned my career choice, my competence, and my wisdom in selecting that couple for licensure. And my choice of toothpaste. *I should have seen it coming*, I thought. But I didn't. It pole-axed me.

By the way, the couple reconciled. Not forever. I got a call from an attorney representing Allison about five years later. They had decided to divorce. They were having—wait for it—a power struggle over who got custody of the child.

That case let me know how fragile couple relationships are and how fragile our therapeutic progress can be. And it showed me that my loss of hope as therapist was profound. Even if it was for only a couple of weeks. I think that experience sowed the seeds of the hope-focused couple approach (HFCA).

The Power of Hope

The HFCA recognizes the power of hope as a healing agent and the power of loss of hope as a disintegrating force. So, as I slowly used my experience in treating couples as an adjunct to my full-time employment as a professor at VCU, hope became the lens through which I evaluated most theories I read about, the training I sought, and the techniques I tried.

Most of what we discuss in this book is how to form, maintain, strengthen, and rekindle hope in our couples. But we wanted to begin by observing that hope is crucial, even for couple therapists.

Jennifer Ripley joined our doctoral program in the 1990s with a keen interest in couple therapy. I found in Jen someone who was a paragon of hope. Where there was a way with couples, she could find it. Even when there wasn't a way, she could help the couples make a way. Her driving energy came from irrepressible hope.

Jen's Origin Story

Okay, I (Jennifer) confess. My plan to *appear* hopeful was a success!

It is easy to trust Ev and his hopeful ideas because they make so much sense. I trusted Ev that leaning into hope provides the best possible foundation to offer a couple who enters therapy. They come to us tired, anxious, lonely, and desperate. Partners fear that they are losing the *one person* who has known and loved them.

As I began training, I was inspired by Ev to be the last person in the therapy room to give up hope. During the last few decades, when I have supervised the Hope lab at Regent University, there have been plenty of temptations to give up hope as we see couples walking in with power struggles, serious past offenses, and mental health problems. Some partners have never *seen* a healthy relationship in their life. Many partners face substantial economic and social exclusion. Partners sometimes are escaping into numbing activities, flirting online with other options, or emotionally shutting down.

Even the triage work of couple therapy is difficult, figuring what to start on first when the relationship is bleeding out all over the waiting room. Not all couples will be ready for the journey. But the journey is a good one, and they arrive in our offices with the courage to face the struggle and a small hope that perhaps we can help create a loving home. In that reality, we have discovered that it helps to have a hope-filled light in dark lonely places.

So, together we have written this book, and we maintain two websites with free resources for forgiveness or hope-focused interventions (www.evworthington-forgiveness.com and www.hopecouples.com). We hope it will provide you hope when (or if) your clients blow up in your face, and we hope it will keep you moving toward a better practice of couple therapy.

Hope-Focused Couple Approach Is in a 4th Wave of Psychological Psychotherapies

Harvard psychiatrist John Peteet (2023) recently discussed the next wave of psychotherapies, which he called 4th wave therapies. He described the evolution of psychotherapy as having developed in three waves.

- 1st Wave (to the 1960s): Psychodynamic therapies, which aim to enhance autonomy and mastery through insight and ego control.
- 2nd Wave (cresting in the 1980s): Cognitive, RET, CBT, family systems (Minuchin, Haley), Gestalt, and traditional behavior therapies (Jacobson & Margolin). They aim toward present-oriented, problem-solving cognitive changes.
- 3rd Wave (1990s, cresting in the 2000s and 2010s): Integrated behavior therapy and spin-offs—ACT, DBT—solution-focused therapy, schema-based therapies, and mindfulness-based therapies. They aim at solutions and emotional-disengagement techniques.

Peteet (2023) said 4th wave psychotherapies aim beyond insight, mastery, conscious action, problem-solving, and disengagement from consciousness. They try to promote value- and virtue-oriented living that results in flourishing and well-being rather than mere problem-solving or solution-focus. They build on the legacy of existential, humanistic, positive psychology, and spiritually oriented therapies, but they differ in not embracing traditional approaches.

He listed some examples of 4th wave therapies. These include derivatives from positive psychology—virtue promotion, character-strength building, happiness and well-being enhancing. Others draw weakly from spiritual traditions (generally with religion removed)—loving kindness-producing exercises, meditation methods, mindfulness disengagement, promotion of dignity, promotion of gratitude, meaning-centered approaches, forgiveness-oriented approaches, humility-oriented approaches, diversity-consciousness including spiritually and religiously informed approaches.

We were surprised to find ourselves surfing the 4th wave. Ev started the HFCA back in the late 1980s, blending hope with virtue, well-being, meaning, forgiveness, and humility! We are glad to see that the HFCA has become more relevant in the last decade.

Reference

Peteet, J. R. (2023) The virtues in psychiatric treatment. *Frontiers in Psychiatry, 14*, 1035530. doi: 10.3389/fpsyt.2023.1035530

Part 1

Framing Interventions

2 Introducing the Theory

Use Five Steps in Operation Hope

No general entering battle—what it often feels like in couple therapy—enters without a grand strategy for the entire campaign. The Imjin War in the late 1500s is known for extreme success and failure strategies. Here's one example.

The war was fought in Korea with invading Japanese samurai and sailors. Japanese warlord Hideyoshi planned to ferry his well-trained military to Korea with a massive naval assault. Fearing the worst, Korean general Shin Rip set up his defenses in a swamp so his troops couldn't quickly retreat. Well, that worked. But it also made them unable to maneuver in battle. (Oops.) To make matters worse, he outfitted them with shorter-range weapons than the Japanese. It was a massacre, largely due to poor strategy.

This book aims to develop your strategy—both your grand strategy and your strategy for battles—and the tactics (flowing from your strategies) that you'll use during sessions. We want to equip couple therapists with the latest effective techniques. Yet, we believe that a grand campaign strategy will help you see your theoretical approach in perspective and improve your ultimate choice of battle-strategies, techniques, and tactical decisions in couple therapy.

If you get nothing else from this book, we hope you will learn this campaign strategy. This is a therapy theory. It is so simple that couples can understand it, even when emotionally caught up in their deteriorating relationship. Also, it is so simple that therapists can retain it, even when struggling with the sparks of a volatile couple conflict or the disappointment of a couple announcing that they don't want to continue after the current session.

It is simple in concept, but the theory is complex and contains many well-developed research-based theories and practice-tested approaches. So, as we move through the book, the simple structure will be fleshed out.

DOI: 10.4324/9781003009382-3

Operation Hope: The Grand Campaign Strategy

Examine Figure 2-1, and we'll talk you through it. First, a word about how the figure is drawn: the five circles are the major steps of Operation Hope. Concentrate on those. The squares are different aspects that make up the major concepts, and we will get into them in the following chapters.

Hope (step 1) energizes two cascades—one for the therapist (steps 2 and 3) and the other for the couple (steps 4 and 5). Hope fuels your, the couple therapist's, choices of strategies. Then, based on the strategy for a particular session, hope provides confidence in your use of particular techniques.

Hope also fuels the couple's change efforts. Especially in the early phases of couple therapy, you will supply much of the couple's hope. Hope is intensely interpersonal and communal. There are many times when we all feel hope is at a low ebb and we need someone to speak hope to us, so we can employ that hope. So, as you provide them with hope, the couple can begin to work at modifying the damage to the emotional bond that underlies their relationship problems. The way that bond is repaired is through engaging in the activities of therapy, as well as the work at home that comes from therapy and the partners' own initiatives. That will eventually, in most cases, yield good outcomes that strengthen the relationship and the partners.

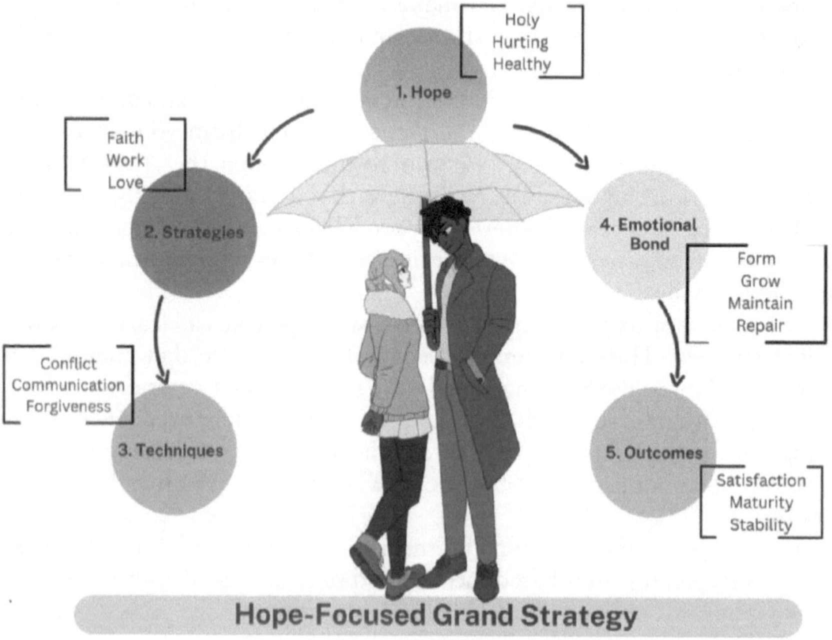

Figure 2.1 Operation Hope: The Grand Strategy for the Hope-Focused Couple Approach (HFCA)

Theory of Treatment

As discussed, there are two cascades. In one, therapists draw on hope to develop a strategy and then use that strategy to target problems. In the other, the couple receives hope from the therapist until it grows into their own experience of hope.

Hope for holy, hurting, and healthy

Step one is built on Rick Snyder's (1994) seminal work described goal-oriented hope as requiring agency and pathways to change, called willpower and waypower to change. Worthington et al. (2015) have added a third component, waitpower, to persevere when change is not apparent. A scale has recently been developed to measure waitpower (Rueger et al., 2023). Over a lifetime, waiting is a very important skill for couples. Partners will become sick or depressed, face grief or job loss, care for newborns or aging parents, or have different goals and needs at various times in a family life cycle. Partners who can "wait it out" through a stage of family life, making the best of their willpower and waypower, often find a future stage of family more easily aligned and peaceful.

Hope resonates with anyone who cries out to the Universe in the night with pain in their relationship. Ask couples when they are especially struggling. What do they do when it's late at night, and they feel it in their bed? Maybe it's a prayer for rescue and a miracle in their relationship from God or the Universe. All human hearts long for something better than this world of pain and struggle. Everyone needs hope for the holy sacred moments alone on their bed, for managing the current hurt, and for facing the fear of a future without love.

The therapist's cascade—a strategy of faith, work, and love

Step two is the cascade that allows therapists to develop an operational strategy to change relational patterns. The strategy has three parts:

1 *Love* is defined as being willing to value and not devalue the partner.
2 *Work* is essential to change. It is defined as putting energy into the relationship. Partners need to invest their energy (and time and emotion) into the treatment for the time they have committed to couple therapy.
3 *Faith* has many objects. These include faith in the partner, faith that change is possible, faith in the relationship, and faith in the therapist's ability to help. Religious or spiritual faith is also an important motivator for religiously or spiritually engaged couples.

The strategy of the hope-focused couple approach (HFCA) is to promote love, work, and faith with couples. Love is at the center. People come to couple therapy because they feel they have lost the love they once had, and so the HFCA uses their language to connect with them. Work is essential to change. When many couples attend therapy, they might hope for "love surgery," for the removal of a troublesome partner, for example, or at least to heal their broken heart instantly. Or they do not expect to change. Many expect to be able to say, "We tried everything we could to save the relationship—even couple counseling." Many couples are double-minded. They want to revive their relationship but also want to run from the pain. Instead of advocating escape, the HFCA engages them with an initial head-on assessment of difficulties and possibilities. Then, it presents them with a feedback session in which (if they are to continue with therapy) they will be asked for an agreement to spend a work-week of 40 hours of work (including in-therapy time) to improve the relationship. This work-week engages them in 20 or more hours of working on their relationship outside the face-to-face therapy time. Finally, faith is promoted. The patients must have faith that the therapist can help them, faith that the partner can change, faith that the relationship is salvageable, and faith in their ability to stick with the couple's therapy until a fair chance at restoration has been given. The most direct test of this strategy was in a five-hour couple-enrichment treatment (Worthington et al., 1997). Couples (n = 51) either met with therapists for hope-focused treatment or received only assessment and feedback. Hope-focused was more effective than the assessment-only control condition in dyadic adjustment, couple satisfaction, and commitment.

The therapist's cascade—techniques that target problems

Step three are the techniques. The Johnsons arrive at your office. Five years of withdrawal and defensiveness have left emotional scars. Malik's doom-scrolling on the internet is impressive. Serena's ability to stay busy with work and children from 4 am to 10 pm and avoid her husband fuels serious anxiety. They sit.

Serena opened. "We hardly communicate any more. Our children are leaving home soon. We don't want to break up once they are gone, but I'm afraid we are headed there. We started to talk about this, but it ended in a fight."

Malik chipped in, "Yeah, we never fight cause we never talk! Our friend said you helped them. We thought coming here was worth trying at least. Can you help us communicate?"

If you have seen a couple like this, you know the path will likely be long. Years of avoidance won't give way to three weeks of communication training.

The Johnsons need to find good techniques that target problems like communication, conflict, intimacy-avoidance issues, and repairing offenses. Research indicates that couples' felt need is likely to be communication, conflict, or intimacy complaints (Doss et al., 2004). Their felt need is important. We take it seriously. Interventions to identify and target those needs are a key step of the grand strategy of HFCA.

In Intervention 2-1, we list ten techniques under which we organize HFCA therapy. Techniques 1 through 5 have also been tested together under the component HOPE—handling our problems effectively. Techniques 6 through 9 have been tested under the component FREE—forgiveness and reconciliation through experiencing empathy.

Intervention 2-1 Ten Techniques of the HFCA

HOPE

1 Assessing and providing feedback—some of which might occur as homework.
2 Interviewing positively—a history helps reframe the relationship in a context that gives more weight to the positive interactions than partners attributed to it.
3 Resolving differences—breaking up old patterns and forming new ones. This includes interventions like TANGO and LOVE, and evaluating underlying interests rather than positions.
4 Assisting in positive communication—using interventions like love bank, date night, listener–speaker, and Positive Active Responding.
5 Encouraging emotional, social, and sexual intimacy—exploring distancer–pursuer patterns, tracking emotional intimacy changes weekly, or finding creative ways to increase intimacy by a half point on a scale of 0 to 10.

FREE

6 Examining alternatives to forgiveness as an antidote to offense—including alternatives like seeking justice, turning the matter over to God, minimizing the importance of engaging in active conflict, tolerating the other's aggravating behavior, forbearing, and accepting.

7 Promoting forgiveness (if desired)—teaching the REACH forgiveness model to one partner then the other, completing a DIY workbook, using forgiveness to forgive a hot-button issue, or participating in a REACH forgiveness psychoeducational group.
8 Promoting reconciliation—teaching reproaches, confessions, homework to write out a good confession to be read to the partner next session, and coaching partners on responses when a good confession is made.
9 Building trust—fostering trusting and trustworthy interactions and gaining anxiety-management skills (that can signal trust).

TERMINATION

10 Consolidating gains—using homework (such as working on a DIY workbook on forgiveness) and creating a "graduation" memorial, then receiving a final report and feedback.

These ten components are how the therapist helps build hope (the underlying currency throughout treatment). All are already evidence-based interventions. Thus, as a clinician, you don't risk being accused of using an "experimental treatment."

The couple's cascade—forming, growing, maintaining, and repairing the emotional bond

Step four is built on the science of attachment. The adult love bond is the primary adult attachment. The similarity with the childhood parent–child bond is uncanny in biological, observational, and self-report research (Burgess-Moser et al., 2016). Attachment style is an individual construct. Two people with secure attachment styles can have a lousy emotional bond between them. But, individual attachment styles are good predictors of successful adult bonds.

Humans move from relationship bond to bond in their lifetime and flourish when in healthy relationships. For most adults, that's a long-term marriage-type relationship.

Part of understanding couples is understanding how they regard the history of their emotional bond and their individual capacities to connect more deeply. New couples are forming their bond. The relationship may end quickly if things go wrong. Sometimes, that is best for both partners early in the relationship. Unhealthy, anxious attachment characterizing one or both partners' styles can lead people to hold onto an unhealthy emotional bond too tightly in a relationship in the early "getting to know you", stage. Not all relationships should grow.

For those who make it past the early stage, the bond grows as the couple learns their strengths and weaknesses. The bond will grow if they find enough similarities to enjoy, and yet some differences for a sense of being well-rounded and individuated as a couple. For instance, Jen is not good at tracking finances, and her husband is great at it, so early in their relationship, they developed an appreciation of differences. Couples get access to each other's brains and abilities, building their bond.

Once the emotional bond is strong, it has to be maintained over time. Ruptures are ubiquitous. Integrative behavioral couple therapy has a brilliant concept. It recognizes that all couples have (some) incompatible differences (Christensen et al., 2020). When stressed out, many couples seem to have one person who uses talk to cope with the stress while the other uses quiet to cope. Those two coping strategies are incompatible! Sometimes, incompatibility can become extremely difficult to tolerate. When loss or trauma enters the family, each partner may feel desperate to survive using their own coping style. This means the emotional bond will probably face damages. The couple will need to repair the bond. Some couples struggle to repair or have weak bonds at every stage. Usually, they are in your waiting room feeling a sense of hopelessness. As therapist, it will be part of your job to hold out hope to get them moving.

The couple's cascade—outcomes of couple intervention

The final step five focuses on outcomes. If you put a group of therapists together in a room and ask them, "What are YOU hoping will happen in couples at the end of therapy?" we bet there will be many answers. Researchers generally choose relationship satisfaction as an outcome measure, which is likely a good "blood pressure" measure of relationship health. Like the doctor checking our vitals, if our blood pressure is elevated, we usually have something off indicating we're sick. The underlying problem, however, may be trust issues, large offenses or many small ones, harsh communication, avoidance of intimacy, lack of consideration for differences, or many other things. Let's focus on three good "vitals" for couples.

First, satisfaction is important. Couple relationships generally will provide happiness or satisfaction in life. Most Westerners especially value happiness as a high goal in life. Those in other cultures may be less focused on happiness but still like to be happy. Second, maturity is important. There should be a sense of growing, maturing, and becoming wiser over time in the relationship. This measure might fit better in Eastern cultures that value the wisdom that comes over time. This is harder to measure, but there are plenty of signs of maturity, like putting aside one's own needs for the sake of the other within a balanced relationship. Third, stability is important. Most couples want the long-term commitment of a stable relationship they can count on to have a flourishing life in terms of children, home, friendships, and extended family.

The Science that Supports Operation Hope

HFCA = HOPE + FREE. Several thousand hours of detailed research on the HFCA have demonstrated the efficacy of its two main intervention components. HFCA is a pluralistic therapy that draws from several approaches to form two main components—HOPE and FREE—that *usually* work. It gives us a starting point to create a grand strategy for treatment instead of guessing or going with our gut in treatment. We can begin with what usually works. Then we can adjust and use creativity to tailor the treatment to individual couples.

HOPE involves assessment, feedback, communication, conflict resolution, and intimacy training. FREE involves explicit training in forgiving and communicating about transgressions in ways that will promote reconciliation rather than rancor. These two components have been tested against each other three times (Burchard et al., 2003; Ripley & Worthington, 2002; Worthington et al., 2015). The main findings have been that HOPE and FREE have different effects. HOPE, which is more communication-based, promotes rapid change but its effects decay. FREE, which assumes that problems will arise but couples can forgive and reconcile, doesn't rise as fast, but gains are maintained. Also, we found that secular versions of the HFCA work as well with religious couples as do religious versions matched to their beliefs, values, and practices.

HOPE has been tested against other control conditions (Worthington et al., 1997), and it has a therapeutic effect on couples. The subcomponents of HOPE have been evaluated also. Findings suggest that work with individual couples was superior to couple-groups. Also, we found that separate assessment and feedback sessions produced a substantial therapeutic effect (Ripley et al., 2002; Worthington et al., 1995).

FREE has been evaluated in numerous treatments. FREE is a forgiveness intervention that can be used with couples who wish to try to forgive. FREE has been used many ways. One way is to separate partners to work on forgiveness and then bring them back together to discuss their progress. FREE intervention helps clients be decisionally forgiven, learn the REACH forgiveness model, discuss an injustice gap, and narrow it through admitting responsibility, offering apologies, expressing empathy for the hurt caused the partner, and making efforts to make amends. All of that happens within the broader context of reconciling.

Reconciling involves four "planks" in a "Bridge to Reconciliation." These involve:

- Decisions about reconciling,
- Discussions about the transgressions,
- Detoxification of the relationship, and
- Devotion to the future progress of the relationship.

Most of the talk about forgiveness occurs within the discussion phase of reconciliation.

The subcomponents of FREE have received a large amount of research, showing them to be evidence-based. The REACH forgiveness protocol with individuals has been tested in over 30 randomized controlled trials (for a review, see Worthington & Wade, 2020). The FREE subcomponents include the value of apologizing in response to reproaches (Miller et al., 2013) and how to respond to apologies and requests for forgiveness (Jennings et al., 2016), both of which have been tested and found to be efficacious.

The HFCA is broadly usable. Its techniques draw from several schools of couple therapy. Yet, we have a developed focus (i.e., hope), strategy (i.e., promote love, work on the relationship, and faith in the partner, the relationship, and the future), and an organizational framework centered around a particular problem-solving focus (i.e., communication, conflict resolution, intimacy promotion, forgiveness, and reconciliation).

The Hope-Focused Couple Approach—Some Recent Advances

Earlier, we said that the approach was largely set by 2014. However, our studies of outcomes, processes, and basic psychological processes on which the HFCA is based have continued since then. Those studies in the last ten years have yielded new aspects while not altering the basic theory or approach. Five findings are most relevant.

First, new clinical methods have been developed. We have included over 100 in this book.

Second, a new measure of "waitpower"—the Persevering Hope Scale (Rueger et al., 2023)—has been developed. Our experience with the measure is that couples are reluctant to report a loss of will to persevere until they bottom out in hope. However, this has not been tested in clinical research. Thus, we suggest caution in interpreting the results if you use it with couples in therapy.

Third, we have conducted three large practice-based studies of therapists in actual practice and their client couples. We found that religious therapists in general couple-therapy practice, often with many religious clients among their caseloads, identify the HFCA as their most-used approach (Hook & Worthington, 2009; Hook et al., 2014). We also found that many people who identified as primarily HFCA therapists used techniques from other approaches and that many therapists who identified with other approaches used HFCA techniques within their practice (Ripley et al., 2022).

Fourth, we followed up on outcomes for over eight years post-therapy for couples. There were still gains from when they entered couple therapy.

Fifth, research on promoting forgiveness has blossomed. The REACH forgiveness method (Worthington, 2006,) has over 30 randomized controlled trials supporting its effectiveness. This includes 24 studies in groups and 7 studies of DIY workbooks, including a multi-nation study involving 4,598 participants (Ho et al., 2024).

Conclusion

The HFCA theory draws on all categories of couple therapy interventions (Lebow & Snyder, 2023), although not every theory of couple therapy. As a pluralistic therapy, it has evidence for good outcomes (relationship satisfaction and stability), supporting its use in both couple therapy and couple enrichment. Thus, it is likely that you might find some overlap with your personal preferences for therapeutic approaches.

One strength of the HFCA is that, from the outset, it has not been merely investigated as a complete approach to therapy. Because it was formulated by drawing on different approaches, we have sought to investigate the effectiveness of different components and their subcomponents that make up the method. You can, to some degree, pick and choose different techniques or modules that fit with your approach to add diversity to your couple therapy techniques.

References

Burchard, G. A., Yarhouse, M. A., Kilian, M. K., Worthington, E. L., Jr., Berry, J. W., & Canter, D. E. (2003). A study of two marital enrichment programs and couples' quality of life. *Journal of Psychology & Theology, 31*, 240–252.

Burgess-Moser, M., Johnson, S. M., Dalgleish, T. L., Lafontaine, M. F., Wiebe, S. A., & Tasca, G. A. (2016). Changes in relationship-specific attachment in emotionally focused couple therapy. *Journal of Marital and Family Therapy*, 42, 231–45.

Christensen, A., Doss, B. D., & Jacobson, N. S. (2020). *Integrative Behavioral Couple Therapy: A Therapist's Guide to Creating Acceptance and Change*, 2nd edition. New York: WW Norton Co.

Doss, B. D., Simpson, L. E., & Christensen, A. (2004). Why do couples seek marital therapy? *Professional Psychology: Research and Practice, 35,* 608–614.

Ho, M. Y., Worthington, E. L., Jr., Cowden, R. G., Bechara, A. O., Chen, Z. J., Gunatirin, E. Y., Joynt, S., Khalanskyi, V. V., Korzhov, H., Kurniati, N. M. T., Rodriguez, N., Salnykova, A. A., Shtanko, L., Tymchenko, S., Voytenko, V. L., Zulkaida, A., Mathur, M. B., & VanderWeele, T. J. (2024). International REACH forgiveness intervention: A multisite randomized controlled trial. *BMJ Public Health,* https://doi.org/10.1136/bmjph-2023-000072

Hook, J. N., & Worthington, E. L. (2009). Christian couple counseling by professional, pastoral, and lay counselors from a protestant perspective: A nationwide survey. *American Journal of Family Therapy, 37*(2), 169–183.

Hook, J. N., Worthington, E. L., Jr., Atkins, D., & Davis, D. E. (2014). Religion and couple therapy: Description and preliminary outcome data. *Psychology of Religion and Spirituality*, *6*(2), 94–101.

Jennings, D. J. II, Worthington, E. L., Jr., Van Tongeren, D. R., Hook, J. N., Davis, D. E., Gartner, A. L., Greer, C. L., & Mosher, D. K. (2016). The transgressor's response to denied forgiveness. *Journal of Psychology and Theology, 44*(1), 16–27.

Lebow, J. L., & Snyder, D. K. (Eds.). (2023). *Clinical Handbook of Couple Therapy, 6th ed.* The Guilford Press.

Miller, A. J., Worthington, E. L., Jr., Hook, J. N., Davis, D. E., Gartner, A. L., & Frohne, N. A. (2013). Managing hurt and disappointment: Improving communication of reproach and apology. *Journal of Mental Health Counseling, 35*(2), 108–123.

Ripley, J. S., Borden, C. R., Albach, K., Barlow, L. L., Kemper, S. D., Valdez, S., Babcock, J., Smith, C., & Page, M. (2002). Providing personalized feedback for marriage enrichment through distance formats: A pilot project. *Marriage and Family: A Christian Journal, 5,* 215–228.

Ripley, J. S., & Worthington, E. L., Jr. (2002). Hope-focused and forgiveness-based group interventions to promote marital enrichment. *Journal of Counseling and Development, 80,* 452–463.

Ripley, J. S., Worthington, E. L., Jr., Kent, V., Loewer, E., & Chen, Z. J. (2022). Community-based spiritually integrated couple therapy: Christian-accommodated couple therapy as an illustration. *Psychotherapy*, *59*(3), 382–391.

Rueger, S. Y., Worthington, E. L., Jr., Davis, E. B., Chen, Z. J., Moloney, J., Eveleigh, E., Stone, L. B., Glowiak, K. J., & Lemke, A. W. (2023). Development and initial validation of the Persevering Hope Scale: Measuring wait-power in three independent samples. *Journal of Personality Assessment*, *105*(1), 58–73. DOI:10.1080/00223891.2022.2032100

Snyder, C. R. (1994). *The Psychology of Hope.* The Free Press.

Worthington, E. L., Jr. (2006). *Forgiveness and Reconciliation: Theory and Application.* Brunner-Routledge.

Worthington, E. L., Jr., Berry, J. W., Hook, J. N., Davis, D. E., Scherer, M., Griffin, B. J., Wade, N. G., Yarhouse, M., Ripley, J. S., Miller, A. J., Sharp, C. B, Canter, D. E., & Campana, K. L. (2015). Forgiveness-reconciliation and communication-conflict-resolution interventions versus rested controls in early married couples. *Journal of Counseling Psychology*, *62*(1), 14–27.

Worthington, E. L., Jr., Hight, T. L., Ripley, J. S., Perrone, K. M., Kurusu, T. A., & Jones, D. R. (1997). Strategic hope-focused relationship-enrichment counseling with individual couples. *Journal of Counseling Psychology, 44*, 381–389.

Worthington, E. L., Jr., McCullough, M. E., Shortz, J. L., Mindes, E. J., Sandage, S. J., & Chartrand, J. M. (1995). Can marital assessment and feedback improve marriages? Assessment as a brief marital enrichment procedure. *Journal of Counseling Psychology, 42,* 466–475.

Worthington, E. L., Jr., & Wade, N. G. (2020). A new perspective on forgiveness research. In E. L. Worthington Jr. & N. G. Wade (Eds.), *Handbook of Forgiveness*, 2nd ed. (pp. 345–355). Routledge.

3 Promoting Hope

Uncover Different Kinds of Hope

Problem: Hope is lost in many seeking couple therapy.
Solution: Promote multiple and complex types of hope.

We love the end of the 1977 *Star Wars, Episode 4—A New Hope*. The Galactic Empire's Death Star has gone operational and has already been used to destroy a civilization. It is about to be used to destroy the base of the Rebel Alliance.

The rebels have virtually no chance of winning this war against the powerful Empire and their star bad-guy, Darth Vader. But they got secret schematics of the Death Star, which show a flaw in its thermal exhaust port leading to the central reactor. It can be exploited if someone flies into the center of the Death Star and photon-torpedoes the reactor.

So, the rebels send a suicide mission to attack the Death Star and its hundreds of fighter ships to divert attention from the only attack that can accomplish the mission, which Luke and a couple of other pilots will launch. They tried to get the rogue smuggler, Han Solo, to join the mission. Han didn't like the odds. He told Luke he would go solo and enjoy the bounty he and his Wookie companion, Chewbacca, had earned by helping Luke rescue Princess Leia from Darth Vader's clutches.

Hope is at a low ebb. But they still have a goal. They have the will to carry their suicide mission out and they know how to fly to make it work. They have goal-oriented hope for the healthy, and they have persevering hope to see it through.

The rebels launch the diversion and the suicide mission. In the battle, the rebel fleet is almost wiped out. Hope is almost gone. They have three fighters left—Luke and two other pilots. They can't see how three fighters can get through.

Then (if that weren't discouraging enough), Darth Vader attacks the three. Boom. Now there are two. Bam. Then one. Only Luke remains with

DOI: 10.4324/9781003009382-4

Darth Vader on his tail, lining up the kill shot. Hope for the hurting is about to go down in flames. But Luke perseveres in what we might call, hope for the hurting—persevering hope.

There seems to be no way out. Luke can only hope for a miraculous rescue. He must turn to what we might call hope for the holy.

Does Luke get his last-minute, just-in-the-nick-of-time miracle? Who blows Darth Vader away? Right. Han Solo. He swoops in and knocks Darth Vader tumbling into space. Help arrived, and Luke's hopes are vindicated. Luke destroys the Death Star. And they live happily ever after. Well, at least until *The Empire Strikes Back* (May 1980).

Three Types of Hope

There are three types of hope. Hope for the holy is hope in a higher power, love, or cosmic justice in the Universe. Hope for the hurting places hope that the pain will be worth it and end in a better outcome due to persevering through a painful sacrifice. Hope for the healthy is hope that accumulated work and building healthy skills and habits will triumph over the obstacles we face.

For people that believe in a higher power, they are rooted in the same thing—putting hope in a trustworthy god. For those who doubt or don't follow a higher power, there is a need to hope for something better—something meaningful and purposeful—that humans can attain. We will look at three concepts that illustrate these three types of hope.

Conceptual Theory in the HFCA (How Hope Contributes to Desired Clinical Changes)

Couples have an *ultimate desired change* of a committed and satisfying relationship for both partners. They want this to last for as long as they live. Yet, when they come to therapy, they are usually demoralized and in low hope.

Couple therapists are crucibles of hope that they distribute to couples. The ladle with which they dispense hope is a therapeutic strategy. That strategy guides specific techniques, each of which is infused with the therapist's hope. As partners respond to the techniques, hope is gained by the partners. They feel that a stronger emotional bond being forged. That stronger bond provides the hope that allows them to experience seven improved outcomes: (a) increased communication; (b) better handling of conflict and better resolution of differences; (c) increased positive experiences of intimacy; (d) addressing hurts and injustices through forgiveness or other means; (e) restoration of trust; (f) reconciliation; and (g) solidifying gains. But how does hope infiltrate these processes?

How willpower, waypower, or waitpower hope contributes to (→) proximal changes

1 Hope → increased communication.

If there is hope, partners will communicate more openly and effectively (i.e., waypower). Successes feed increased willpower or agency. When communication problems recur, after partners thought they had those communication difficulties resolved, persevering hope (i.e., waitpower) is needed to keep channels of communication open. Also, better communication can trigger hope, which encourages continued efforts to improve communication.

2 Hope → better handling of conflict and resolution of differences.

Similar reasoning can feed better resolution of differences. Hope inspires people to try to manage conflict better. Hope generated by successful resolution of differences, in turn, generates renewed efforts to resolve even more differences.

3 Hope → enhanced intimacy.

Intimacy is fed by hope and also feeds hope. But intimacy involves an additional consideration. Some people fear intimacy. Few people are anxious about communicating. Most people want to resolve differences. But many people fear being close to and known by their partner—especially if they have been in hurtful conflict. They can feel exposed and vulnerable if they are better known. Therapists need to tread cautiously in advocating for vulnerability. Some people simply are toxic and will use the partner's vulnerability to inflict more damage.

4 Hope → more forgiveness.

Research repeatedly shows that forgiveness is correlated with hope (Washington-Nortey et al., 2022). Interventions to promote forgiveness produce more hope in the relationship. Hope that the relationship can improve also makes it more likely that partners might be willing to forgive.

5 Hope → increased trust.

Hope is helpful to the couple relationship. It increases the sense of safety and the belief that the relationship can be improved. This hope increases trusting and trustworthy exchanges between partners. Often, in the early stages when hope is scarce, the therapist must bravely model what it means to be trusting and solidly trustworthy.

6 Hope → reconciliation.

Reconciliation is a restoration of trust when trust has been damaged. It involves relational repair that proceeds from the increased trust and produces more trust. Importantly, trust can only increase if partners perceive each other as at least trying to be trustworthy.

7 Hope → solidified gains.

When partners have hope, they are more likely to believe that hard-won gains might continue and grow. Think about a case you have seen. Perhaps a couple initially fears losing their relationship and motivation to change. Self-sabotaging behaviors can torpedo their hope. Partners try to repair injury inflicted in nasty fights. But they keep bringing up the argument and reminding their partner of past hurts and ugly exchanges. As a therapist, you must discover how to correct their criticism without yourself sounding critical. Point them to how to act in the future rather than dwell on how they have been acting.

The March from Proximal Changes to Ultimate Change

We suggested that *techniques* that change proximal targets of therapy, like communication or intimacy, are guided by a *strategy* of faith, work, and love. The strategy springs from *hope*. The successful use of the strategy and techniques will, in turn, lead to forming a strong *emotional bond*. That will produce improved *couple outcomes* of stability, maturity, and satisfaction. As you see, hope is clearly the center. Hope generates changes and changes generate hope.

Reference

Washington-Nortey, P. M., Worthington, E. L., Jr., & Ahmed, R. (2022). The scientific study of forgiveness, hope, and religion/spirituality. In E. B. Davis, E. L. Worthington, Jr., & S. A. Schnitker (Eds.), *Handbook of Positive Psychology, Religion, and Spirituality* (pp. 361–377). Springer. Open access. https://link.springer.com/book/10.1007/978-3-031-10274-5

4 Employing Strategies for Love
Faith Working through Love

Problem:	Couples have lost faith, work, and love in their relationship.
Solution:	Employ strategies that target faith, work, and love as effective means for relational change.

A successful couple relationship is satisfying, stable, and mature. Such couple relationships require faith, work, and love. We use these terms because they are part of the common vocabulary of couples who have relationship strains. Thus, using such terms helps us easily connect with them. We don't need to spend an hour explaining our terminology. They appreciate the plain talk of a therapist.

Faith

Faith is confidence in whatever is hoped for, based on evidence. Don't be put off by the term. We are not talking about religious faith here. Faith has an object. We have faith in many "somethings." Those "somethings" provide targets for intervention.

Faith permeates all life. Think how much faith it takes to venture out onto the highways in our car. Will other cars keep to their lanes? Will they drive responsibly? Will they run stoplights? Will they speed? Will they drive aggressively? And will I do all those things and uphold my civic responsibilities regarding driving? Our lives hang in the balance.

Faith is needed in all relationships, but couple relationships are especially predicated on faith. Perhaps you have seen couples question their partner's overall intent. They wonder, if their partner is out to get them? Do they love me? Will they prioritize the marriage? Will they cheat? Are they just trying to make me miserable? Can I have faith in their trustworthiness—to do the taxes, manage the kids responsibly, hold a job? If my partner says they will change, can I count on a good faith effort?

DOI: 10.4324/9781003009382-5

Faith is intimately involved in therapy. Can I have faith in the therapist to treat our relationship with value? To be fair? To maintain confidentiality? Will the couple therapist use science-supported methods? Will they respect my values?

If we, as therapists, detect a weakness in faith, that tells us what we should do. For example, if we see that we've done something that the couple does not agree with and their faith in our ability to help seems impaired, we must address this therapeutic rupture in the session.

A couple Jen saw in therapy appeared to be just working on communication. This should always be a clue that no one is "just" working on communication.

Here's what happened. The woman had a drunken make-out session with someone else when the couple had temporarily broken up. She was remorseful. He had said often that he had forgiven her. As they talked about whether to go to a party that weekend, the man suddenly flew into a jealous rage about her fidelity. He had no faith in her character, and his distrust was always just below the surface. That weakness in faith completely blindsided the woman—and Jen.

If the couple has a crisis in faith at week 5, which is fairly typical, they might be losing faith that therapy can help. We can use that crisis in faith to show them that progress in therapy often happens in three phases (Howard et al., 1993). Use psychoeducation to get this across (see Intervention 4-1). In the initial phase of therapy, called *remoralization* because the couple is usually demoralized at the outset of therapy, the couple often has surging hope, which is often deflated by an unanticipated crisis. The second phase, *remediation*, is usually where symptoms are resolved. The third, *rehabilitation*, is where functioning is reforged and stabilized.

Intervention 4-1 Education About Couple Therapy

In the early stages of therapy when faith, work, and love are low, infuse hope through good psychoeducation about the normal course of treatment and expectations for couple therapy. Consider adding written ideas to your website, creating short videos explaining couple therapy, or making a digital training platform with visuals and voice to catch their attention and shape their thinking. This investment also will likely increase couples who "stick" in the early stages of treatment when dropout is highest. Here are possible psychoeducational topics.

1 The three phases of couple therapy (remoralization, remediation, and rehabilitation; Howard et al., 1993) are evidence-based. Create a handout or

webpage with education about these three phases. This alerts couples to what often happens in therapy (normalizing it), and it increases your credibility if they run into some hiccups.

2 The systems-run-downhill concept can help them understand the importance of homework.
3 Explaining your approach to couple counseling and why you think it works can help couples understand the principles behind your techniques and interventions. For example, check out a blog on our website (hopecouples.com) called "What is hope-focused couple counseling and why does it work?" After the intake, we ask couples to access that (or print it out for them).
4 "Is this couple ready to commit to therapy?" is a major question in early treatment. Education on the process can answer common questions that partners hold that can impede commitment. These include things like, "Will my partner change?" or "Are there situations where couple counseling isn't a good idea?" or "One of us is reluctant to attend, what should we do?" We have also created a blog on our website to address these questions.
5 If you give any homework to all (or almost all) of the couples you see, then education about that homework can be standardized.

Work

To improve a system, work must be supplied (see Intervention 4-2). In physics, work is putting energy into a system. Without the input of energy, any system tends to chaos. The second law of thermodynamics, which we're sure rolls off the common tongue, says that in a closed system, disorder will inevitably increase over time.

Intervention 4-2 Get This Across—In Couple Therapy, Work Is Essential

At the start of therapy, it is important to characterize the therapy work as real work. Partners not experienced in therapy can be unrealistic about the amount of work needed to create lasting change, which will take some months of sustained effort. The work will take time.

Metaphors and examples are helpful to normalize the expectation for couple therapy work. For example, finances will dissipate if we don't put effort into managing them. If we don't put the energy into cleaning the house, it will become dirty. If we don't put energy into maintaining our car, it will eventually break down.

Initial expectations about work required to succeed in couple therapy

Couples can agree with the abstract concept that work is needed to succeed in therapy. Yet they often can't put that abstract belief to work. When asked how long people think therapy should take, they usually say they'll be done in three to five sessions. Frankly, it's like the old comic panel by cartoonist Sidney Harris. Two scientists are looking at a whiteboard. One scientist has derived equations, one systematic step after another. But there is a missing step. Beside that missing step, a handwritten note says, "Then a miracle occurs." This seems to be the way most people treat psychological interventions. Step 1 is to enter therapy. Step 3 is to emerge with no problems. Step 2—what happens in treatment—is blank, with a note that says, "Before the third session, a miracle occurs." Part of helping people succeed in therapy is to provide information. Here's what's crucial. (1) Therapy usually takes longer than you expect. (2) You are not guaranteed 100 percent probability of success. (3) You'll need to work. (4) A lot.

Use homework to leverage the amount of work partners do

Not all types of psychotherapies use homework. Generally, cognitive-behavioral, cognitive, and behavioral psychotherapies believe homework is necessary to help people change. Much research has shown that those approaches with homework have better outcomes than the same approaches without homework. In addition, if you assign homework, make sure you follow up to ensure the partners did it.

Other types of therapy, like emotionally focused couple therapy, focus on in-session change with little homework (Thet, 2022). Some types of psychotherapies do not advocate homework. Therapies without homework tend to take a bit longer to achieve the same results.

Despite being an approach that draws from many types of therapy, some that do and some that don't favor homework, we have found homework helpful from the standpoint of our clinical experience. We think therapy sessions make a big impact. But they don't always. Ev recounts a session that resulted in a couple crying, embracing, and laughing together. "This was life-changing, they claimed as they left." Ev secretly exercised his narcissistic fantasies that Oprah would phone him demanding to see the videotape of the session and show it (with the couple's approval, certainly) on prime-time daytime television. The next week, Ev went into the session to see what the next steps would be after the life-altering session of the previous week.

"So, how was the week?"
"Great," one of the partners said.
"Did you all put into practice some of the insights you had last week?"
Silence. Stringing out uncomfortably long. Then . . . "Uh, can you refresh our memory on what we did last week?"

Good thing Oprah didn't call in mid-week.

Such experiences erode the confidence that many of our sessions are ever life-changing. To increase the likelihood of change, we can use the other 167 hours of non-session time. Good homework can demonstrate faithful commitment to the partner, which increases their bond, redirect them from negative patterns to experience more positive ones, and direct them toward their goals with practical, sensible techniques they can do on their own seems to work, and couples like it.

For some couples, "homework" is a four-letter word. Getting their cooperation requires some skill. We have found this approach (see Intervention 4-3) to work well.

Intervention 4-3 You Just Have to Do a Week of Work

The couple therapist has presented the treatment plan and negotiated any changes with the couple. Let's say they agreed to a 12-week intervention period. Here's the way the conversation might unfold.

Couple: Therapist — We will be meeting 12 hourly sessions starting next week and ending four months from now. I've already told you the research showing that you'll probably need at least that much time for sessions. But we cannot hope to accomplish in one hour per week—twelve short hours—the changes you need after eight years of marriage, with the last three being filled with conflict and some emotional distancing from each other. I'm afraid you'll need to commit to some additional time working on your marriage outside of the therapy sessions. Are you willing to do that?

Husband: What are we talking about here? I've got lots of commitments at work and other things.

Wife:	Of course, I expected him to say this. I told you he wasn't committed to changing.
Husband:	That's unfair. Just because I have lots of irons in the fire, . . .
Therapist: (interrupts)	Let me be more concrete. I think you all have invested eight years plus your two years of dating and engagement into the relationship. I assume that investment is not something you want to lose just from giving up a few hours to focus on your relationship. I'm just talking about one work-week on the marriage—40 hours.
Wife:	That doesn't sound too bad.
(Silence, then) : Husband	Can we count the 12 hours in session?
Therapist:	Sure. Forty hours, counting 12 hours in session and 28 hours of dedicated time working directly on your marriage outside of sessions, practicing things that make your relationship more positive and enjoyable.
Husband:	Sounds doable.
Wife:	Sure.
Therapist:	So, can I get your commitment that you are willing to spend that 28 hours outside of therapy working with dedication on bettering the marriage?
Both:	Yes.

A work-week of homework might not sound like much. So, couples almost always agree. But the facts are, few clients ever actually do that much homework. If we can get people to do 28 hours of homework on their relationship, we have dramatically increased their likelihood of staying engaged throughout the week. Here are some homework interventions you might recommend (see Intervention 4-4).

Intervention 4-4 Great Homework Interventions

Certain types of tasks lend themselves to homework more than others. Partners can:

- Practice the skills learned in therapy.
- Reflect on the insights they gained in the sessions (such as doing worksheets).

- Monitor their behavior by completing logs or self-assessments to inform them whether they are progressing.
- Broaden their knowledge about treatment or aspects of it by watching YouTube videos, TEDx talks, and podcasts can be inspirational and educational.
- Plan positive time together and make room in their schedules for having such time.
- Write letters to themselves or their partner.
- Go on romantic dates to increase their emotional bond.

Use session reviews as work to help partners process what happened in sessions

After-action reviews can be used throughout couple therapy. They are structured ways of reviewing sessions. They take a few moments each week, but they're worth it! They are especially important when emotional experiences are evoked. You can use our Reflective Processing Worksheet (see Intervention 4-5) or adapt your own method. You'll probably only need to use this once or twice. Partners learn what to do after they've been through a structured exercise a couple of times, and sometimes they will replace this structure with a discussion about what happened. The worksheet will help partners learn it—and it fits with our philosophy of "making change sensible" by using tangible materials to supplement discussion.

Intervention 4-5 Reflective Processing Worksheet[1]

This is a couple-conversation starter worksheet. We hope it will encourage you to discuss what happened in the session or in a homework activity.

From your perspective, what happened today (or just now) in your session? Write a brief summary.

Is there something important to remember from this session? Write a summary.

How can you connect what you learned in this session to what you are learning about your relationship and how you are changing overall?

If something is important to you, commit and share it with your therapist and partner. This week, I will . . .

Love

Love can be defined in many ways. Lebow and Snyder (2022) suggest that all couple therapy approaches have distinct theories of love that are explicit or implicit. For some, love lies in growing the couple's friendship; for others, in the attachment; for others, in how partners think and feel about their relationship; for others, the broader historical or cultural context; for some, sexuality; for still others, deep intrapsychic needs and capacities to connect. Some theories stress peak experiences and intensity of connection; others stress steadiness and order. A best-selling book says love is a language (Chapman, 2010). Most approaches speak of multiple layers of experience but emphasize one lens—spotlighting love, connection, and health.

We think of love using a simple-to-grasp definition. *Love* is valuing the partner and not devaluing the partner. When asked, most couples who seek therapy say,

- "We have lost our first love."
- "Our problem is that love has faded."
- "Our goal is to restore love."
- "If we just still loved each other, we could deal with the stresses in our marriage."
- "When we were in love, things were great."

Because couples use "love"-language, we do, too. It builds a stronger therapeutic alliance and connects us with couples. It aligns our goals with their goals. Love is valuing the partner and not devaluing the partner (see Intervention 4-6).

Intervention 4-6 Love that Values the Partner In Action

This intervention is super-flexible. It focuses the couple on positive, valuing, loving actions they have taken and can take in the future. Love in action could be:

1 Make a list of loving actions each partner does but does not tell the partner. Then, do a few of those things during the week. Try to catch each other doing them. Reveal what they did before the next therapy session and see if they were "caught."
2 Do a five love languages® quiz (https://5lovelanguages.com/quizzes/love-language) and use that for ideas to do in the partner's primary love language.

3. Create a list of things each partner appreciates that the other person has done for them in the past. Refrain from saying, "But you don't do it anymore."
4. Write down 50 things about their partner that they appreciate and love. Frame it as a gift.

Strategy—Promoting Faith, Work, and Love

So, we have a general therapeutic strategy—to promote faith, work, and love to build more robust emotional bonds between partners. We keep this in mind as we design and carry out therapy. But ideally, we want partners also to learn the strategy and use it. We hope they will think, how do I have faith in my partner, the therapy, the future? How can I put more productive energy into the relationship? How can I value my partner? If I'm devaluing my partner, can I stop doing that? Each of the interventions we select is aimed at one of these three strategic legs supporting the seat to create a stable resting place for couples—a stable emotional bond, which is the topic we turn to next.

Note

1 BOND Intervention 19-1. Reflective Processing Worksheet (Ripley & Worthington, 2014).

References

Chapman, G. (2010). *The Five Love Languages: The Secret to Love that Lasts.* Northfield Publishing.

Howard, K. I., Lueger, R. J., Maling, M. S., & Martinovich, Z. (1993). A phase model of psychotherapy outcome: Causal mediation of change. *Journal of Consulting and Clinical Psychology, 61*(4), 678–685. https://doi.org/10.1037//oo22-006x.61.4.678. PMID: 8370864.

Lebow, J. L., & Snyder, D. K. (Eds.). (2022. *Clinical Handbook of Couple Therapy, 6th ed.* The Guilford Press.

Ripley, J. S., & Worthington, E. L., Jr. (2014). *Couple Therapy: A New Hope-Focused Approach.* InterVarsity Press.

Thet, C. (2022, July 11). *What's Different About Emotionally Focused Couples Therapy Homework?* Thrive Couple and Family Counseling Services, www.thrivefamilyservices.com/emotionally-focused-couples-therapy-homework/

5 Using Therapy Techniques

Make Change Sensible

Problem:	They make progress in session but falter on their own.
Solution:	Make change sensible.

It never ceased to amaze us. Numerous couples can yearn to repair damage to their relationship, stay engaged with couple therapy, be eager to learn, and apparently be in love. They leave a session on conflict negotiation or communication smiling. Yet before they get to their car, they are arguing. Again!

For years, that was a puzzle. How could that happen? It didn't happen every session. But when it did, it threatened the couple's progress and discouraged couples and therapists. What were the critical cues that led to these post-therapy arguments?

A Detective Story and a Clinical Science Story

We felt like detectives. Okay, we were not Hercule Poirot-type detectives, with the (points to the head) "little gray cells" coalescing to yield a logical answer, despite all the red herrings offered in a typical 53-minute counseling session.

More than a few times, though, it seemed like those therapeutic failures occurred after particularly insightful sessions. That, somehow, didn't seem to make sense. How could a couple's insight into their relationship lead to *failure* in couple communication?

Supervision is a great laboratory for scientific progress—not a controlled experiment. More like the early phase of science. It was like the physicist Tycho Brahe, whose name tumbles out unbidden at social gatherings. I'm sure.

Brahe was an interesting character. His nose was chopped off in a youthful sword duel. But that didn't prevent him from sticking his false nose into

DOI: 10.4324/9781003009382-6

understanding the planets' motion. Between 1570 and his death in 1601, Danish astronomer Brahe made systematic observations of the planetary motions. Observation is the first stage of science. After Brahe died, Johannes Kepler took Brahe's observational data and applied mathematics. He discovered that the data did not fit the "received" science of the day. That anomaly launched the scientific revolution. Our observations weren't of the level of Brahe's, but we couldn't keep our noses out of couples' business either.

We observed that when couple therapists and couples talked with each other about good and bad communication or attempts to resolve differences, they were often energized. Yet, great insights did not always lead to practically applying the ideas in the real world Was the problem our intervention, the partners' perception, or the partners' application?

We felt that the answer lay not in what was taught. Nor in what was applied. The problem was couples' perceiving what was said differently. Like our two eyes that can observe the same thing but have slightly different perspectives, the two partners *often* held different perspectives. Because they were so excited by what they *took to be* the good ideas, they often tried to try to persuade their partner of the truth as they perceived it.

The question, we thought, was, "How can we as therapists reduce the likelihood that the partners develop different perceptions of what they learned?" Our solution: Maybe we could help couples remember the session more similarly to each other if we did not rely solely on talk. Rather we used solid objects in space and time to supplement what the therapist could convey through talk. We called this making change sensible—able to be sensed.

How Might "Making Change Sensible" Work?

One of the interventions Ev had adapted from an early filmed demonstration by Salvador Minuchin (1974) for his Structural Family Therapy was what would later become popularized by Steve de Shazer (1985) as scaling. In the early 1980s, Ev developed a way of promoting intimacy using these ideas (see Ripley & Worthington, 2014; Worthington, 1989; see Intervention 5-1).

Intervention 5-1 How to Do Sensible Scaling with a Couple

1 **Set up the physical analogy.** When couples come to a session to work on increasing intimacy, the therapist asks the partners to get up from their chairs and imagine that the room is a scale of intimacy. "How emotionally close or distant do you feel *right now?* Position yourselves across the room from each other to accurately represent that closeness. Zero intimacy

would be standing on opposite sides of the room and facing away from each other. Perfect, ten-point, intimacy would be both partners hugging in the middle of the room."

2 **Partners try to arrive at a mutual perception of their intimacy.** Let's say that they arrive at level three (fairly emotionally distant but not cold toward each other). They might have to negotiate to arrive at an agreement.
3 **Deal with the dynamics.**

   - If they did not agree on the state of intimacy, even though they were willing to "agree" so that the session could move forward, the therapist might point out that they seemed to be in a power struggle about who has the say. Their power struggle and "agreement" have been illustrated in a way that cannot be later denied. They were trying to position themselves physically and had to come up with a physical solution, not just a solution based on talk alone.
   - Or—depending on the clinical judgment of the therapist—the therapist might note how they at least came to a working agreement. And that is a good sign that they can at least work together when they value the goal.
   - If they could not even "agree" on intimacy, the therapist might ask one person to stay stationary and the other to move, showing her perspective. Then, the other is asked to stay stationary, and the partner moves showing his perspective.

4 **Have the couple arrive at a mutual perception of their ideal intimacy.** Discuss differences in ideal closeness. Many couples have less problem agreeing on how much intimacy they are experiencing at present than on how much they should experience in the ideal state. The emotional distancer–pursuer pattern is often revealed in this intervention. The pursuer wants more closeness than does the distancer, and when they try to show their ideals simultaneously, it often looks like a distancer–pursuer interaction acted out in real time. The pattern is illuminated!
5 **Partners reposition themselves to indicate their current feelings of closeness or distance.** The therapist usually mentions that the recent interactions might have shifted their feelings of closeness. They might reposition at, say, a two. They transition from standing to chairs at that point.

6 **Talk about something that will make them feel closer.** They are directed to talk about something that will bring them closer together. Many power dynamics can be revealed in that interaction. Let's say, though, that they felt particularly close when a miscarriage occurred and they pulled together.

- When the therapist senses they have become emotionally closer, the therapist stops the interaction and has them reposition their chairs.
- Respond to the reaction. Because the therapist has "made" them feel closer, one or both will likely react and do or say something to distance themselves again.
- The therapist has them move their chairs again to signify any change.
- As they continue to discuss their hopes for more intimacy in different types of intimacy—emotional, sexual, intellectual, social, and recreational—the therapist continues to mark shifts in immediate closeness by asking them to reposition their chairs and then discuss why they think their closeness shifted as their discussions progressed.

7 **Draw the lesson explicitly.** By the end of the hour, the point is clear. The partners have it in their power to move closer or more distant as a couple by the way they interact. While this could have been communicated verbally, partners likely disagree about the session's point or whether it was valid afterwards. But when their changes in felt closeness were able to be sensed (i.e., sensible), they cannot disagree with their power to create more distance or closeness within the couple dyad.

Varieties of Ways to Make Change Sensible

Moving the partners around in the physical space is only one of many ways to make change sensible. The point is that conversation alone is easily misremembered. Conversation plus tangible, able-to-be-sensed, physical manipulation is more than doubly helpful.

References

de Shazer, S. (1985). *Keys to Solution in Brief Therapy.* W. W. Norton.

Minuchin, S. (1974). *Families and Family Therapy.* Harvard University Press.

Ripley, J. S., & Worthington, E. L., Jr. (2014). *Couple Therapy: A New Hope-Focused Approach.* InterVarsity Press.

Worthington, E. L., Jr. (1989). *Marriage Counseling: A Christian Approach to Counseling Couples.* InterVarsity Press.

6 Strengthing the Emotional Bond

Focus On What Really Makes Couples Satisfied and Stable

Problem:	Emotional bonds may have never formed well, or have weakened over years of disconnection.
Solution:	Promote emotional connection with couples, not listening skills.

An early implicit theoretical idea in relationship science was that relationships have problems because of poor communication. Misunderstandings seemed so salient during couple breakdowns and conflicts that this seemed logical! Most couples who enter therapy say they need better communication to heal. Thus, historically, much effort sought to find how communication went bad. Then therapy tried to correct or avoid communication flaws.

What Seems Logical Isn't Always True

John Gottman (1994) suggested that one marker could predict whether couples' relationships would disintegrate in the next four years— the ratio of positive to negative communications of less than 5 to 1 during discussions of disagreement predicted relationship dissolution. Bad news: Unhappy couples were more like a ratio of 0.8 to 1. Yikes!

The logical—but it turned out incorrect—therapy intervention was that therapists could help low-ratio (say 1:2 or 1:1 or even 2:1) couples by simply getting them to increase their ratio of positive to negative interactions. Therapists built interventions to promote more positive interactions during discussions and down-regulate negative interactions. Those are great ideas, but . . .

The problem is that correlation is not causation. Poor communication (during conflict negotiations and at other times) was indeed

DOI: 10.4324/9781003009382-7

correlated to how good a relationship was. But poor communication was not driving the bus.

The Emotional Bond

By the early 2000s, most therapists had abandoned the idea that increasing the positive-to-negative ratio could improve a relationship. Couples couldn't keep it up. Not even therapists can be consistently so positive. In their own relationships. It's just too hard. This just-try-harder intervention was an abject failure. By 2010, a new conception—one based on the cause of a good relationship, not trying to remove symptoms of a bad relationship—had swept through couple therapies. To improve the relationship, you need to strengthen the emotional bond between partners.

What this emotional bond is, of course, is thought of differently in different approaches to couple therapy. The base of the bond is similar to adult attachment applied mutually. Attachment is a psychoanalytically informed concept that John Bowlby originated (Holmes, 2014). As such, it is inherently an individual experience. Thinking of each person's attachment style is helpful and provides targets to promote secure adult attachment in each partner. The general assumption would be that if each individual has a secure adult attachment, the dyad must have a secure emotional bond.

Family systems theorists boldly raise their hands and beg to differ. If your parents were terrible to you as a preschooler, are you doomed to a lonely life of anxious or avoidant attachment as an adult? We know many cases where this is not true. Furthermore, adult romantic relationships are opportunities for healing poor attachment. (However, they also can be ways that perpetuate childhood patterns.) Generally, family systems theories might expect that most couples in which partners each had a secure attachment style would develop a secure emotional bond *between* the partners. But systems have a way of being unequal to the sum of the parts.

How Likely Are Strained Emotional Bonds?

So, times of strained emotional bonds might arise and might become self-perpetuating even though, in general, the two partners have secure early attachment styles. Such strains and even ruptures in the emotional bonds might occur for many reasons. For example, a situational strain can bring out the worst in each partner. A simple misspeaking can trigger a deep insecurity. The intrusion of a third party (for example, a friend, a new baby, an in-law with healthcare problems requiring aid, or, of course, an infidelity) can disrupt comfortable patterns of couple behavior. Adult attachments are unique opportunities for secure, anxious, or avoidant attachment *between* two people. These stressful situations can trigger early or adult insecure attachments. But also, emotional bonds can be disrupted while leaving both partners' adult attachments intact.

Therapists know that the therapeutic alliance is extremely important to the success of all types of therapies. Generally, we like to think that we, as therapists, have worked through personal issues to the extent that we are pretty secure in our adult attachments, even though we might have had much to deal with in our families or origin. Yet, we are all too aware that with almost every client we see for an extended time, there are times of rupture of the therapeutic alliance. Suppose we see a client for 20 hours of individual or couple therapy. Is it your experience, like ours, that (on the average) we might experience one or more therapeutic alliance ruptures—usually minor ones, but not always?

With our own experience as background, think of couples with 168 hours of life to live each week. They might spend 55 hours sleeping, 50 hours working and traveling to work, 10 hours alone in sports or physical activity, and up to 25 hours on electronic devices. That still leaves 18 hours that they might spend doing things together (co-action), communicating intimately (including sex), and even doing things alone but in each other's presence (distancing). What are the chances that a rupture occurs in the emotional bond during those 18 hours?

Remember, couples have to share resources, responsibilities, and stressors—which in therapy we don't have to do with clients. Is it any wonder that even satisfied, happy couples have ruptures in their emotional bond?

How Can We Help Couples Strengthen Emotional Bonds?

Tasks as bond

Some tasks must be done or distributed to make a relationship function. Those tasks often are odious and emotionally draining. Those tasks include child-rearing activities and, with sandwich-generation couples, can also include elder care responsibilities.

In the hope-focused couples approach (HFCA), we take tasks seriously. Managing tasks is a major part of an intervention affecting emotional closeness that we call CLEAVE (see Intervention 6-1). Disagreement and misunderstandings can occur over task division, performance, and expectations. These rupture the emotional bond, although usually they are small but can accumulate. Ruptures must be dealt with productively.

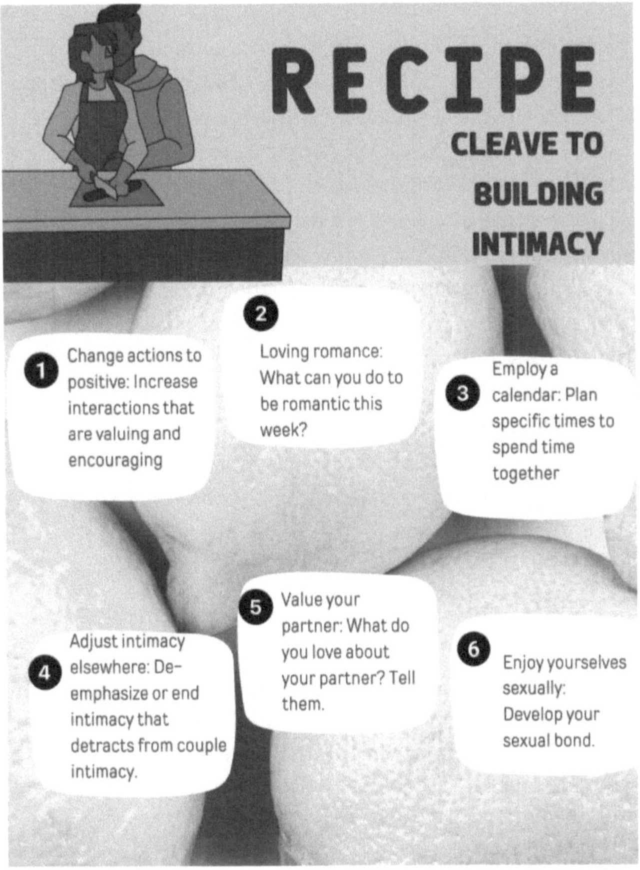

Figure 6-1 Practical Recipe of Actions to Build Intimacy

Intervention 6-1 CLEAVE to Bond[1]

This intervention is really six interventions in one. It works well as homework or some in-session activities. CLEAVE is an acronym to aid the couple's recall of what you talk about in session. They can use it to create specific goals for each category of improving their bond.

- C = Change actions to positive. Do things that bring positivity into the relationship. It might be things like gratitude, fun activities, reading together, watching YouTube videos together, or laughter. Ask your partner what they prefer.

- L = Loving romance. The flame of romance is important in relationships. Small or big actions can show romance. Discuss past romantic activities to come up with ideas.
- E = Employ a calendar. Adjust your schedule to spend more time with your partner. Pick a time for positive interactions. Keep that date. Show you care.
- A = Adjust intimacy elsewhere. It's easy for other things and people to steal time from your relationship. Review your schedule. Consider whether you have let other things intrude on your intimate relationship. No one can spend all their time with their partner, but you can identify obstacles that might be hurting your intimacy.
- V = Value your partner. Look for observable and meaningful ways to show that you value your partner.
- E = Enjoy each other sexually. Sex frequency and activities can be different for each couple. Discuss and work together towards enjoying what you do, when, and how.

Goals as bond

The goals of the relationship are also important to the functioning of the partners. In the HFCA, we pay close attention repeatedly to partners' hopes, dreams, and goals for themselves and the relationship. We ask about those in the assessment, again in the first actual therapy session, further within therapy, and as we near termination.

In any hope-focused approach, hope will rest in those dreams, hopes, and goals (see Intervention 6-2). Often, partners put their relationship on automatic. Inevitable miscues happen. In our voice-to-text functions on phone, text, and email, auto-correct can completely botch our written communication relative to what we intended to say. The same can happen when our relationships are on automatic. Even if we are vigilant about the relationship, we cannot pay close attention to every little thing. Thus, auto-correct miscues are likely. These cause ruptures (usually small) in the emotional bond; like ruptures in tasks, they must be dealt with productively.

Intervention 6-2 Tell Me a Secret—Share Your Dreams

Much research indicates that people develop intimacy through sharing vulnerable and important ideas, values, and experiences and having others respond well to the sharing. Direct couples to share something about their day, life stressors, and dreams that they think their partner might not be fully aware of. Direct them to ask open-ended questions and give full attention to their partner as they share.

A more structured version of this intervention is the "36 questions that lead to love" (Google it). These questions were created by attachment theorist Arthur Aron, especially to bring people together to share dreams, hopes, and fears. As a teaser, the first question is, "Given the choice of anyone in the world, who would you want as a dinner guest?" These questions open couples to build bonds by sharing needs, deep values, and previously unexplored parts of themselves. This can help couples build or rebuild bonds.

Retailers and social media creators understand this. They have created love cards, discussion-starter cards, and online posts with many questions to spark open dialogue.

Emotional connection as bond

Relationships form an emotional connection. That connection is affected by the level of disruption in the emotional bond due to miscues in tasks and goals. But it is also affected by other aspects of a relationship. Personality differences can irritate. The optimist and pessimist who become romantic partners will feel tensions in their emotional bonds. So will the extroverts and introverts, the verbal and silent processors.

Emotional connections are sometimes more fragile than we would like to believe. When couples seem well-matched in emotional connection, it seems more a gift than an application of wisdom. In the HFCA, we spend lots of time on bond. That effort is about repairing ruptures, but importantly, it also involves helping couples attend to and strengthen the emotional bond (see Intervention 6-3).

Intervention 6-3 Attend to the Emotional Cues

Therapists have a superpower through our training in attending to clients' non-verbal and vocal emotional cues. In session, we watch closely as clients are buffeted by their emotions.

Many partners lack awareness of the emotional cues they communicate or perceive in their partner. Partners can look for all the usual suspects: tone of voice (tense, relaxed, raised), word choice (subtle, extreme, subdued), pitch (low and quiet, high), facial expressions (sad face, stoic face, pleasant smile), body language (closed, open, aggressive), and eye contact (engaged, minimal, none). Becoming more aware of emotions can be a powerful way to dig underneath the content of discussion to the emotional meaning and valence.

We offer this warning. We have not found this to be productive with couples who regularly attack each other. They often use their observations as attack weapons, further damaging the relationship. Unhappy but stable couples might find this useful.

Summary

For the HFCA, we look to that positive emotional bond as our target on which we focus the lasers of specific treatment techniques. To inform those techniques, we will discuss principles of couple therapy within the next chapter, which ends this first part of the book.

Note

1 This intervention was originally presented in Worthington (2005) *Hope-Focused Marriage Counseling.*

References

Gottman, J. M. (1994). *What Predicts Divorce? The Relationship Between Marital Processes and Marital Outcomes.* Lawrence Erlbaum Associates.
Holmes, J. (2014). *John Bowlby and Attachment Theory.* Routledge.
Worthington, E. L., Jr. (2005). *Hope-Focused Marriage Counseling: A Guide to Brief Therapy, rev. ed with a new introduction.* InterVarsity Press.

7 Applying Principles of Couple Therapy: Find the Essence of Helping Couples Change

A Baker's Dozen

Problem:	Couples can be like raging elephants in therapy. It's hard to stay focused.
Solution:	Use the 13 principles to guide your work.

Principles can guide much of couple therapy. We admit candidly that much of couple therapy is more about emotion, experience-based intuition, and enduring wisdom than about rational principles. Nevertheless, if we begin by principles, at least we can be intentional about deviating from them on the basis of informed clinical judgment.

Thirteen Principles

So, here we state 13 principles that we think are important in doing couple therapy. In the final chapter, we will reflect on lessons learned to supplement and complement these principles.

Principle 1: Be positive

The hope-focused couple approach (HFCA) is a positive approach to helping couples that uses positive psychology, without being positive psychology per se. Incorporating positive psychology interventions is a real plus in our practice because the field of positive psychology has been committed to evidence-based practices. Therefore, we can usually use interventions from positive psychology with confidence that they work for many people.

Positivity applies to the demeanor of the HFCA therapist, which is positive but not in a namby-pamby, saccharine-sweet way. The therapist promotes hope. Yet the therapist realizes that hope is caught as much as taught. Recall that there are three kinds of hope, and persevering hope

DOI: 10.4324/9781003009382-8

during times of abject suffering is not optimistic, light, and carefree. The therapist must mirror the mood of the partners to connect so that hope can be transmitted. Our therapeutic attitude is, "This is painful and difficult, but we are going in the right direction. You as a couple have done hard things before, and together, we can do this next step of relationship repair."

Principle 2: Use principles of practice informed by clinical science

Relational science informs couple psychotherapy. Our approach to treating couples needs to be consistent with clinical intervention science for couples. Most basic relationship science and neuroscience is based on measures of how couples (usually not clinically troubled couples) *are*. How couples usually function is the start of intervention research, but it is not enough.

Principle 3: Be patient-responsive

At the end of the first quarter of the 21st century, this is probably the main principle for helping couples. Therapists who are not perceived to be responsive to their clients will not be in business long. Patient-responsiveness includes being empathic toward the partners and their struggles.

Most couples come to counseling months or years after the negative patterns are established, despite Oprah's advice to seek help before the problems worsen. They usually don't expect much from couple therapy. Negative outcome expectations can be overcome. Seewald and Rief (2023) found that the therapist's warmth and competence positively combat negative outcome expectations. Perceptions of therapist competence contributed slightly more to the change in expectations than did warmth, but both mattered.

We are reluctant to state what we all know: We need to establish a working alliance early, and we need to repair damage to it when it occurs (for a meta-analysis, see Eubanks et al., 2018). Setting up a great working alliance with two conflicting partners is the genius of couple therapists everywhere. Here are three ways to be patient-responsive. Assess the couple. Assessment is a great way of establishing a positive understanding of a patient-centered relationship—as long as the assessment is seen as necessary, usable, and not burdensome. Then, check in often (and always when an issue arises) about what is happening. Finally, collaborate with the partners in designing and carrying out their treatment.

Principle 4: Focus on hope

Every intervention you make should be tied (at least in your mind) to increasing hope in the couple. While you don't want to burden yourself with a formal evaluation of each intervention, you will benefit if you run through your mind the question, how does this promote more hope or lessen hopelessness? You'll almost unconsciously be asking yourself other questions at the same time. Does this intervention promote work on the relationship? How does this promote love that values the other partner? Does this intervention promote faith in each other, the relationship, or the therapy process? But keep hope foremost.

Principle 5: Prepare for provocation

Partners don't usually set out to provoke you. It just seems like it sometimes. Partners will dump problems on you, sabotage progress, erupt in hot chaos that explodes in sessions, and fail in their goals. When couples fail, it can seem like a direct challenge to your competence as a couple therapist. In our experience supervising dozens of students, such provocations will often bring a supervisee to our door for extra help or support!

When such provocations happen, they are stressors. They trigger stress responses. That means you may experience emotional flooding. Your sympathetic nervous system arousal threatens to downshift you from rational thinking to emotional reactions. With experience, though, you've no doubt developed some effective ways to cope with your own emotional flooding—calming yourself, disengaging from the surface emotion perhaps by making yourself a curious observer, or becoming more task oriented. If you reflect on what works for you, you can teach those coping mechanisms to supervisees who can teach them to their couples.

Principle 6: Base treatment on early assessment

Assess first. Then stop and discuss an agreement to do therapy. Not everything meaningful can be measured, and not everything we measure is necessarily meaningful. We need discernment. Generally, objective measurements will help you. The feedback from the assessment positively affects the couple, preparing them to agree to treatment objectives that you might suggest, enhancing their view of you as a careful expert, and informing initial treatments, just as ongoing assessments will inform whether to continue with treatment plans or make slight (or more drastic) modifications. A treatment plan is, after all, just a plan. "No plan survives first contact with the enemy," says war theoretician Carl von Clausewitz (2008) in his book *On War*. So, we need flexibility.

We must stay open and humble. It is tempting to see all clients as being similar, so, we can easily err in trying to shoehorn couples into plans that have worked with other couples. We have a general treatment plan. That's what this book is about. Yet, we MUST not impose this on the couple. We must integrate it with our unbiased assessment of the couple. And then we must develop our treatment plan collaboratively with the partners.

Principle 7: Always have a treatment plan

Treating a couple is like writing a book. Okay, this just might be on our mind because we are, uh, writing this book. But hang with us to see the similarities.

1 The pressures of time and resources tempt us to cut corners. *Maybe we can "wing it,"* we might think. The couple will never know what we didn't do (that is, plan carefully).
2 We gather basic data before we write or before we counsel.
3 We "outline." The treatment plan is the outline from which we work with the couple.
4 Our organization is tentative. It will change as we go along. Our treatment plan almost always needs tweaking. Sometimes redoing altogether.
5 We write a proposal, which details the outline and fleshes it out, and it clears up things like who the audience is and what we want to accomplish with the book. Similarly, when we present our tentative treatment plan to the couple, writing it down clarifies it.
6 We write the first draft, which will likely differ from the proposal in organization and ideas. New ideas will come, and we must keep revising the organization and main points. We are always learning in our couple therapy.
7 We work on subsequent drafts. As the entire book takes shape, we revise our understanding of the early chapters. We might have to go back and correct things that seemed to be "givens" earlier. One thing is certain in book writing: revision is not done, until the book is printed.
8 We write the book's closing with a powerful finish. It rethinks the initial chapter and guides readers to different futures than they might have anticipated initially. A wise master teacher once said, "Good teaching disturbs and then confirms." It disturbs the learner's idea of the status quo. Dissonance stimulates learning. But good teaching sets the learner back safely on the ground, yet on a higher plane with renewed vision. Good couple therapy does the same. It shakes people out of their unilateral problem-focus, aims them at hopes they might have given up for dead, works with them to reach those hopes, and lands them safely with the renewed hopes in their relationship's ability to live happily without self-destructing.

Principle 8: Include homework as (perhaps) the vital part of your treatment plan

The couple makes the treatment their own when they take it home. Talented individually oriented psychodynamic psychotherapists can sometimes lead patients to such insights during a session that keeps them engaged all week. Some master couple or family therapists can also have such transformative effects without assigning homework. Yeah! Unfortunately, Ev and Jen are not those super-charismatic therapists. Sadly, we must say that few of our trainees had that super-charisma either. But that does not mean we are doomed to a single hour each week. If we can engage partners in work outside the session, the effects of the couple therapy can permeate those other 167 hours of the week. So, for the masses of therapists, let's put effort into designing homework that is not just busy work, but keeps partners engaged all week.

Principle 9: Have a goal of integration as client and couple outcome

Our goal is mature clients, couples, and families. By "mature," we mean that the relationship and the partners understand what they had not understood before, can create and pursue reasonable goals, can control impulses and reactivity with curiosity and calmness, and can translate this into a satisfied and committed long-term relationship. We are tempted to add that world peace is achieved, which is a tongue-in-cheek way of acknowledging that this list is aspirational. Sometimes, we admit, survival is our goal in working with some couples. But, on good days, our dreams and hopes for couples exceed merely helping them (or us) survive another day.

Principle 10: Relationship is our lever, the problems are the fulcrum

Our relationship with the couple is vital. We must connect and stay connected. Ruptures in connection must be quickly repaired. The couple's relationship levers their healing. We noted that the cause of a good relationship is the ability to form, maintain, grow, and repair a strong emotional bond between partners. Thus, making this bond stronger is our target to help partners change their relationship. We must encourage partners to suspend moral judgment of each other's behaviors, especially when actively judging each other. Partners are helped to cultivate digging for COAL. COAL is an acronym for curious, open, accepting, and loving. Sometimes, this requires a lot of digging into the humanity of each partner. Quality COAL is not found in strip mining, which scrapes the surface of their behavior. Rather, they need to get down to their basic values, dreams, hopes, and practices to act on the virtue that they have built over their lives.

The therapist's presence helps the couple find the courage to face the feelings that they have no future, persist in persistent hope, and commit to trying to make a different future than they saw when they came in. The therapist's presence is a portal. A portal is a faster way, a wormhole, into a different place, time, or dimension. Couple therapy is a faster way to a transformed relationship than the partners might forge on their own.

Principle 11: Our method—process past problems and practice for the future

Psychoanalytically informed treatments look to resolving past problems as the key to present and future happiness. Solution-focused therapy guides couples away from past (or even present) problems in small steps today that will help them be much happier in the future, having reached their dreams and hopes. We see value in connecting past, present, and future. We believe it is vital to understand the present and the past (to some degree) to develop an effective treatment plan for the future. So, we begin with an assessment of the history and current state of the couple. This gives the couple confidence that we are treating them personally instead of running an impersonal program on them.

Couples are often excited, enthusiastic, and open to making changes quickly at the beginning of therapy. So, we like the quick engagement in early sessions afforded by solution-focused techniques. But as we work on symptom reduction, we think it is vital to balance handling present problems through better communication, conflict resolution, and intimacy and understanding, with understanding, how those problems developed. Near the end of therapy, most couples want to learn and practice forgiveness as they seek to reconcile. At the end of therapy, we want them to focus on the past weeks and enumerate the learning they experienced. In the final assessment and feedback, we focus the couple on where they are going and what they can do in the future to make it more likely to maintain the gains they worked so hard to build.

Principle 12: Our plan is to heal couple's downhill cascade

John Gottman has identified the four horsemen of the apocalypse for relationships (Gottman & Silver, 2015). He has found that criticism is responded to with defensiveness, which leads to more criticism. At some point in the downhill cascade of the relationship, the partners seem to stop focusing on behaviors of criticism and defensiveness. They change how they think about their partner, viewing them with contempt. That fundamental shift usually signifies a worsening of the relationship that can lead to stonewalling (i.e., trying to withdraw from the fray emotionally) or war (i.e., entering into the fray with full engagement).

Let's think about the four horsemen differently. Some strategies are attack strategies. These involve criticism, contempt, conflict provocation, and response. All of those create chaos. They attack the emotional bond by actively seeking to disrupt it. Other strategies are defensive. These involve defiance, defensiveness, and disengagement. Defensive strategies confound connection. They can destroy the emotional bond while seeming to try to preserve it. We plan to illuminate the painful process and bring order into the chaos by providing more mature, healthy alternatives to attacking or withdrawing. We actively undermine their defenses with love and humility exercises.

Principle 13: Treat tornados as both distractions and opportunities

Disasters disrupt treatment. Each week, the couple can come in with a new disaster (or several). We call them tornados. They are cyclical patterns of pain—EF-1 through sometimes EF-5—that distract from facing problems head-on. In fact, after a particularly good session with tears, hugs, and apologies, you can predict for the couple that their painful patterns will try to re-establish themselves. Tell them to watch for a tornado in the next week. Those tornados are real disruptions in the life of the couple. But there are also disruptions in the couple's treatment, unless the therapist can stick to the treatment script and tie the disasters to the treatment plan. Your task is to incorporate the painful tornados into the treatment plan. This is where your genius and experienced savvy come in.

Looking Ahead

The rest of the book will show how we put these principles into practical operation. We use the HFCA, not because we are attempting to somehow lure you into using the approach whole-hog, but because the principles are most concrete and easy to grasp as they are applied within a particular approach. Therefore, we will walk you through the method from the first contact to the end of the termination session.

References

Eubanks, C. F., Muran, J. C., & Safran, J. D. (2018). Alliance rupture repair: A meta-analysis. *Psychotherapy*, *55*(4), 508–519.

Gottman, J., & Silver, N. (2015). The Seven Principles for Making Marriage Work: A Practical Guide from the Country's Foremost Relationship Expert. Harmony.

Seewald, A., & Rief, W. (2023). How to change negative outcome expectations in psychotherapy? The role of the therapist's warmth and competence. *Clinical Psychological Science, 11*(1), 149–163. https://doi.org/10.1177/21677026221094331

von Clausewitz, C., (2008). *On War*. Princeton University Press.

Part 2

Interacting Hopefully

8 Building Hope with HOPE

Handling Our Problems Effectively

Problem:	Relationship education and skills are not sufficient to create change.
Solution:	Therapists craft experiences with relationship skills to create hope, which opens pathways to improved emotional bond.

Many new therapists come to our training with two faulty ideas: (1) Helping couples learn relationship education and skills will cure their relationship problems; (2) The couple already has hope that change is possible. Both of these assumptions are incorrect.

If education were enough then the thousands of self-help couple books would have caused a surge in happy relationships. That has not happened. The effectiveness of self-help couple relationship books is limited. You might think if couples learned good listening skills, or other relationship skills, that would solve their problems. It won't. Most people know how to help their relationship. They just can't do it under the pressure of interacting. Intuitively couples know this to be true.

That is why hope has bottomed by the time they enter couple therapy. They have tried books or online relationship advice, talked with friends or clergy, and prayed to the Universe. Yet the threat of losing their bond is so noxious that they are even willing to try (gasp!) couple therapy. As therapists, we should take their discouragement seriously.

HOPE and FREE: Skills and Forgiveness

There are two legs for the hope-focused couple approach (HFCA) to stand on, HOPE, or handling our problems effectively, and FREE, forgiveness and reconciliation through experiencing empathy (Worthington et al., 2015).

DOI: 10.4324/9781003009382-10

We'll discuss HOPE in Parts 2 and 3 of this book. HOPE, which fuels the building of emotional bonds, consists of skills-heavy methods that tend to produce rapid changes that lead to hope. Conflict reduction, communication, and building intimacy help stabilize couples who need to know they *can* improve. During the initial re-moralization phase of therapy, where energy is high, these are a perfect match to redirect weary couples. Also, many couples believe that their problems are due to poor communication. So, working on that fits with their expectations and builds a stronger working alliance.

The other modality of the HFCA is FREE, which drives the repair of emotional bonds. We'll discuss FREE in Parts 4, 5, and 6 of this book.

Skills are needed by couples, and skills require practice. If we were going to run a marathon, we could read books about how to run marathons, have friends encourage us to run marathons, and have coaches whip up our emotions and motivations until we were straining at the bit to run marathons. But we might not get to the starting line before we'd be sucking wind. Unless. Unless, we actually trained and practiced marathon-running skills and girded ourselves for the challenges of Heartbreak Hill.

Couples can learn some new skills, and use them effectively, if they are simple, sensible, and targeted to the problem they are facing. All of the HOPE interventions are created with that assumption. Yet it's important to remember that skills are not enough. If the skills don't improve the bond, that will discourage the couple.

Skill Trainings Are Exercises to Engage Partners

New therapists often believe that relationship-skill education is the key to change. It is easy to think that skill education teaches troubled couples how to turn their marriage around.

If only it were that easy.

Consider this. How much are we are actually teaching this Google-savvy population about communication and conflict resolution? Do we really believe that our clients have not heard about the importance of empathy, active listening, reflecting content, using I-statements instead of you-statements, not criticizing, and not treating the partner with contempt? Relationship education is everywhere in common culture—YouTube videos, podcasts, TEDx talks, SNL skits. In our couple therapy, we teach couples little they don't know. They *know* the right answer to the question of what they need to do. Much of it is common sense. If you yell at your partner and emotionally push them away, they will not want to have sex with you tonight. Duh. Everyone knows this. Yet people yell and push all the time.

What we do in couple therapy is not teach new stuff so much as provide structures to help them do what they know but can't seem to call to mind at the right time. Or, even if they do think of it, they can't do it in the heat of a discussion; we try to find a structure that can help.

But wait! We still teach the skills, even though they are part of the common culture. Why? Because by practicing them, couples break up negative default patterns and thus stop damaging their emotional bond. Instead, they:

- Demonstrate that they care enough to change by doing what does not come naturally in the midst of an argument.
- Slow down their rampage.
- Stop the tornado cycle of conflict more quickly.
- Change the structure of their patterns of normal everyday interaction, which allows maintenance of the improved emotional bond.

And, yes, on occasion, they actually do add a skill to their behavioral repertoire like the Alligator Intervention (see Intervention 8-1).

Intervention 8-1 The Alligator Intervention (Or How to Respond When Your Partner Snaps)

Partners might snap at each other in the office. Or partners will report that it happened during the week. To help couples note their default automatic pattern and practice new patterns, we can characterize habitual snapping as a quick, automatic, angry emotional response. Here are five ideas to help the alligator-snapping couple:

1 When alligators snap, quickly apply first aid. Remind partners that quick reaction kept humans alive for eons. The same brain that allows you to quickly kill a spider crawling up your leg or save a toddler from falling off a swing, also snaps at the partner. Reframe the snap as a protective, fearful, spider-killing, toddler-saving super-power instead of an insensitive mean act that reveals a deficient character. Frame the problem this way: "Snaps happen." But it's what you do next that matters.
2 Alligator snaps are predictable. When we are tired, hungry, stressed, hurt, or taxed we are more likely to snap at each other. Most couples can identify when they are likely to snap. When an alligator comes to the surface, don't taunt it with a juicy chicken! Learn when not to try to solve problems. Brainstorm times during the regular schedule when difficult discussions, persuasion tactics, or complex activities are best postponed.

3 Never swim alone. Not all snaps are fatal. Some just nip. Partners can be wonderful resources for soothing the alligator because, well, everyone is an alligator. Help partners consider ways they have soothed each other in the past. How do they solicit needed support? Because a couple's brains are deeply connected, soothing the partner has a direct positive effect on the soother and soothee. If the snap is a minor "ouchee," it's okay to support a snapper. When the snap is injurious, though, that is a time to get out of the swamp—distance and disengage.
4 Time out for alligators. Everyone can remember a nighttime fight that looks silly in the morning. If only a brief time out could have happened, the silly fight could have been avoided. Sometimes time is needed to allow for the stress hormones and defenses to recede. During a safety time out, partners can work intentionally to soothe themselves and down-regulate their emotions. Characterize short-term disengagement as a healthy choice. Some couples mistakenly think they need to resolve all their problems immediately. Also, using a time out to rehearse their comeback speech or plan how to hurt the partner won't end in a hug. Just more snapping. Partners can think of ways to bring the alligator back to calm.
5 Be kind to the alligators. Creating a home characterized by understanding and grace for occasional normal snapping is healthier than a perfectionistic home. Occasionally a partner will have more serious anger or aggression problems. If partners are unable to practice alternatives to snapping in your office or fail to improve in homework, then some evidence-based anger management interventions might be needed.

Understanding HOPE

HOPE produces hope, which is the fuel to improve bonds. The experiences in therapy and homework that improve communication, conflict resolution, and intimacy contribute to the experience of hope. Hope opens pathways to forming, maintaining, growing, and (to some extent) healing bonds. All of that work promotes hope, the essential ingredient to change in relationships. This is why we say HOPE promotes hope.

Virtually all approaches to couple therapy agree that success in couple therapy is about helping couples strengthen and repair the emotional bonds between them. Conflict is often the most visible problem in couple therapy. So, it is what couple therapists often see first. In the remaining chapters of Part 2, it's important to keep in mind that relationship skills are not the real avenue to change. The relationship experiences inherent in the skills are a way to promote hope and stronger bonding. Our first step in HOPE, is figuring out with the couple what we need to change. So, we begin with assessment.

Reference

Worthington, E. L., Jr., Berry, J. W., Hook, J. N., Davis, D. E., Scherer, M., Griffin, B. J., Wade, N. G., Yarhouse, M., Ripley, J. S., Miller, A. J., Sharp, C. B, Canter, D. E., & Campana, K. L. (2015). Forgiveness-reconciliation and communication-conflict-resolution interventions versus retested controls in early married couples. *Journal of Counseling Psychology*, 62(1), 14–27.

9 Understanding the Couple's Problems and Goals

Use Assessment Efficiently

Problem:	The first few sessions set the pace for couple therapy.
Solution:	Excellent assessment, feedback, starting homework right away, and routine outcome monitoring assessment will be state-of-the-art couple care.

If we don't get off on the right foot with a couple, we are running uphill in a three-leg race. Blindfolded. The first session is all-important. Obviously, this gets couple therapy moving in the right direction. Without the remainder of therapy, a great start will fizzle. But without the great start, therapy will be a real slog.

We believe assessment and feedback are the keys to successful couple therapy. So, in this chapter, we are providing guidance in more detail than we usually do.

Our usual way of working with couples is to agree ahead of time to an extended assessment session (usually two sessions) prior to making any commitment to couple therapy. Clients complete scales ahead of the session. Couples have a two-hour assessment interview, which also includes videoed discussions and sometimes individual time to address red-flag issues or pathology. Then, the therapist takes the videos, scales, and interview results and prepares a report and tentative treatment plan. However, everything is based on a collaborative, patient-responsive model of therapy. Collaboration happens in a one-hour feedback session. We present the results of the assessment and tentative plan. We then discuss it and agree on the treatment plan and treatment duration for actual therapy.

This chapter will offer you seven keys to an excellent assessment for couples. These involve communicating what the hope-focused couple approach (HFCA) offers and responding to couple preferences, conducting

DOI: 10.4324/9781003009382-11

a welcoming intake, using a couple-interaction video demonstration, setting up the first homework, providing excellent but efficient written feedback report and treatment plan using hope principles, deciding whether HFCA is right for the couple, and using routine outcome monitoring throughout treatment. Let's jump in.

Why Assess Couples Up Front and Provide Explicit Feedback

There are many reasons to assess and provide feedback at the outset of therapy. We will discuss each below.

Up-front assessment and feedback contribute to couple improvement

Up-front assessment and feedback take about three hours. This has been investigated and found to be perhaps the single most powerful intervention in couple therapy (see Worthington et al., 1995).

It can engage reluctant partners in therapy

Often one partner is the advocate for therapy but the other is more reluctant. Therapists are always looking for a win–win solution to such conflicts. That win–win is found not in compromise or in supporting the partner who is seeking therapy; it is found in meeting the underlying interests of both partners.

At the outset, we have partners agree to assessment and feedback, not couple therapy. We say that we'll make clear recommendations about whether we see therapy as needed by the end of the feedback session. By shifting from deciding about therapy to deciding about assessment and feedback, the partner advocating for therapy is supported because the other partner is working with a therapist. But by making a commitment only to assessment and feedback, the reluctant partner is not "losing." Reluctant partners can often agree to an objective person helping with the relationship and offering expert opinions on the course of couple therapy or ideas for relational growth.

It is part of what prevents premature termination

Swift and Greenberg (2014a) offer practical strategies that can prevent termination before couples reach their therapeutic goals. In a continuing education course, Swift summarized eight evidence-based strategies (www.tzkseminars.com/psychotherapy/). Four of those strategies are employed at the outset of therapy, and we'll digest each of them. Much of their book is based on individual therapy, but their recommendations agree with the strategies we've used.

It sets up a collaborative frame from the outset

Most therapists today have given up the doctor-knows-best approach to therapy in favor of a collaborative, patient-responsive approach. So, we use a collaborative framework that most therapists and clients are comfortable with today. By getting partners to give you their views on the relationship through written scales, enactments of their communication, and discussion, you engage them in providing specific information about their perspectives on the relationship. By providing feedback and seeking collaboration, you engage partners in planning their own treatment.

The feedback, in particular, is educative

When partners complete assessments and see their numbers, especially when compared to norms, the result is educative. Just completing scales can be therapeutic. It encourages reflection. But the feedback to couples about what happens in couple therapy is educative more broadly, and it sets realistic expectations for therapy.

It guides partners in understanding their roles, the therapist's role, and the approach

Swift and Greenberg (2014b) recommend that therapists provide role induction. By this, they means that the therapist should ensure that clients understand their treatment, the roles and responsibilities of therapist and client, and expected outcomes. Clients often have misinformation or are unsure about things like cost, what can be talked about, whether advice will be given, or whether they will practice what they learn out of session. Actually, role inductions are ongoing. They take place whenever needed but always at the beginning of therapy.

They recommend that the therapist provide such information through a website or pamphlet. He also recommends a brief orienting video that walks the client virtually through the reception process, the waiting area, the therapist room, and aspects of how therapy might be conducted. These suggestions have much evidence supporting them. Swift et al. (2023) meta-analyzed 17 studies that used role induction. The dropout rate was 64 percent less than when no role induction was used. Outcomes such as what to expect in therapy, immediate engagement with therapy, client ratings of the therapeutic alliance, and masked observer ratings of clients' readiness for therapy were also superior in clients receiving role-induction information.

Assessment engages preferences for couple therapy

In the feedback session, the therapist negotiates with partners which preferences can be incorporated into couple therapy. Patients have choices. See Intervention 9-1 regarding education for clients about their preferences. We incorporate a second strategy to reduce the likelihood of premature termination—consider client preferences or educate them about your parameters. Swift et al. (2012) meta-analyzed 28 studies and found that client–therapist dyads that were mismatched on preferences were 79 percent more likely to drop out. In 51 outcome studies, matched clients were more likely to have positive treatment outcomes.

Intervention 9-1 Educate Couples about Preferences Intervention

These parameters help couples know what they are signing up for, if they choose to engage in HFCA with you. This could be a simple handout for couples. It clearly communicates what you, or your practice, can provide and what limitations exist. For example, the HFCA has specific parameters.

In your couple therapy, here is what usually happens. You can have input if you disagree with any of these. HFCA:

- Focuses on a specific goal to help you improve your emotional bond through relationship exercises and experiences.
- Uses assessment and feedback for 2–3 sessions; after that, you decide whether this treatment meets your needs.
- Uses routine outcome monitoring to weekly monitor progress. This helps clear roadblocks more quickly.
- Tends to be 8–18 sessions in duration. Sessions are either 60 or 90 minutes, usually weekly. Sometimes sessions can be offered in more intense formats, such as a double-session intervention to foster quick change.
- Offers relational skills to raise hope for a better future and relationship bond.
- Engages in repair through forgiveness, empathy, understanding, and compassionate responses to each other.
- Involves work at home, both individual and couple.
- Collaborates with you, but the therapist offers exercises and ideas for therapy.

- Focuses on your relationship, not on one partner as deficient.
- Is more present- than past-focused.
- Engages the emotions of the relationship.
- Challenges partners to be humble and reconsider their perspective.
- Supports the diverse needs of couples.
- Seeks to keep sessions productive; the therapist may interrupt partner interactions at times if critical or defensive in sessions to replace them with more helpful interactions.

Partners may prefer different things. One partner may want weekly behavioral therapy with homework and an active therapist. The other may want insight-oriented reflection. One partner may want a male therapist, and the other partner may want a female therapist. You want to be attuned to whether, if they disagree on therapist preference, they are using that issue as a power struggle.

Either way, such disagreements can have therapeutic upsides. When you work with conflicted couples to help resolve conflicts, you might use, as the HFCA advocates, the Harvard Negotiating Project's Getting-to-Yes program (Fisher et al., 2011). At the core of this method is realization that the positions people take are often irreconcilable. Yet, underneath the positions are interests that lie under those positions. Those interests often can be met by a creative win–win solution that does not lead down the primrose path of trying to compromise on two incompatible positions.

Plan for termination from the beginning

In the feedback session, the therapist provides accurate information about how long couple therapy might be—based on the average for all couples and individually tailored to the particular couple. The third strategy for minimizing premature dropout is to plan, from the outset, for appropriate termination (Swift et al., 2023). Swift et al. (2011) found that most clients entering therapy believe they will only need to attend for 3 to 5 sessions. In fact, in 13 to 18 sessions, about 50 percent of people fully recover (Swift et al., 2011). By correcting unreasonably optimistic expectations, dropouts will be lessened. Swift and Greenberg (2012) meta-analyzed 669 outcome studies, involving almost 84,000 clients in individual psychotherapy. They found that time-limited treatments had fewer premature dropouts than did open-ended therapies. Ask couples to estimate the number of sessions they believe will be necessary to reach their hopes and dreams for successful couple therapy. If partners guess 3 to 5 sessions, you can cautiously agree and then disagree with them You might say, "It's possible you will reach your goals in 5 weeks. Do you mind if I share some research with you?" If the couple agrees, you can say,

> In over 600 studies, the average number of sessions it takes for half of the people to reach their goals is between 13 and 18. So, you might be correct that it takes many fewer sessions for you all to reach your goals. But maybe I could suggest a middle ground. If you are willing to enter into couple therapy, what if we planned for about 12 sessions? But what if we build in a re-evaluation point at about session 6? By then, you might feel that you have reached your goals, but you might find that you are closer to the average of 13 to 18. If you decide at session 6 to continue, then by session 12, you might feel satisfied with where you are. But we also might re-evaluate again at that point, and you might even want to change your expectations again. We would agree to stay flexible and keep an eye on your relationship as we move through therapy. In the end, if you decide to go on with couple therapy, it's up to you as to how many sessions we plan.

Of course, these are averages. One of the things we as therapists are certain of is that there is no average couple. Couples get better in one, three, twelve, eighteen, or twenty-six sessions. Or they don't. Some get worse, and therapy is their gateway to divorce. So, the preparation of an individualized plan for the couple is absolutely crucial.

Educate couples about how change can happen

The fourth recommendation to minimize dropouts is to educate partners about typical patterns of change (Swift et al., 2023). In 1989, Worthington (1989) noted that progress in couple therapy was often substantial at first, but a dip in satisfaction occurred around session 4 or 5 for many couples. He recommended having a preprinted graph showing that decline as a way of "talking couples off of the ledge" of giving up. The preprinted graph normalizes backsliding. Howard et al. (1993) found that most clients enter psychotherapy demoralized and low in hope. They found that two to four sessions constituted the re-moralization phase of psychotherapy, characterized by rapid improvement as hope is re-experienced. But, often around session 5, a relapse was normal. Howard et al. also noted that between sessions 5 and from 8 to 12, symptoms begin to decrease (i.e., the remediation phase), but often patients saw that as reason for termination. Yet, for people to regain normal functioning often took up to 18 sessions for half of the people and for the other half, termination took longer.

Promote hope

The fifth strategy for minimizing dropout—seek to promote hope—can be practiced throughout therapy, not just at the outset (Swift et al. 2023). However, there are things that the therapist can do early in treatment. To help partners' willpower to change, focus on partners' strengths rather than on problems. Reinforce strengths in the feedback report, by complimenting them for successful completion of tasks, and by interpreting task completion as willingness to work on the relationship. Jen often uses the Values in Action brief character strengths survey, created by Martin Seligman (Seligman et al, 2004) and easily found in a Google search. Instead of partners filling it out on themselves, they complete it on their partner, which provides information to include in the feedback report on what strengths their *partner* notices in them. To help partners' waypower to change, seek to convince partners that the treatment they might be about to commit to will be an effective way to improve. This can include describing a persuasive treatment rationale, success rate, evidence supporting the effectiveness of the treatment, and therapist anecdotes about patients who succeeded.

What We Want to Accomplish in the Initial Sessions

There are two important goals for initial sessions. We want to help partners conclude that therapy is a safe space with a safe therapist and that it is more important to try to change than to determine how they can blame their partner for problems. These two major goals are intertwined. But for ease of communication, we are going to separate the specific objectives for the sessions into two goals—relationship-focus and hope-focus. Here are some important tasks to accomplish.

Build a working alliance

All approaches to couple therapy aim to build a great working alliance with the couple. The alliance keeps the couple wanting to return to therapy because they trust the therapist. But a good therapeutic alliance is not just relational. It creates a safe space for the couple to air their stories and try out solutions.

When most couples attend therapy, they are fighting for survival—of their relationship, their self-concept (as a romantic partner), their self-esteem, and sometimes their psychological integrity. In stress-and-coping terms, they have encountered multiple stressors and have appraised the relationship as threatened. Almost all partners who attend therapy have their stress reactions cranked up to full volume.

Create safety

Because they see stress everywhere, it is our job as therapist to create a safe space. Safe spaces give people a place to breathe, to reconnect with oneself, one's partner, and one's reasons for being in the relationship. The therapist fosters safety by being personable and trustworthy. Friedman (2017) emphasizes that the therapist must have a non-anxious presence, bringing that safety to couples models and setting the tone for what the future of their relationship can be like. Peacemakers know this. When President Jimmy Carter invited Menachem Begin of Israel and Anwar Sadat of Egypt to peace talks in 1979, he invited them to the bucolic Camp David. He drew them out of the normal negotiating rooms and day-to-day routines. Even that was not enough to promote good peace talks. In fact, Carter confessed in some of his memoirs that the talks had failed. Sadat was packing his bags. Carter went to his living quarters at Camp David and took pictures of his grandchildren. He talked with Begin about peace for their grandchildren. Only then was Begin able to agree to even meet again. But the real turnaround happened when all three men met informally the next day. All three trotted out pictures of their grandchildren and agreed that they did not want their own grandchildren to grow up in a world marked by the conflicts of recent years. Through that safe place, talking about something they valued, they finally began to move toward what became the Camp David Accord.

The therapist enters through the open door without forcing his or her way in

We do this by not contracting for therapy at the outset of the intake, as we've explained above.

The therapist establishes ground rules

These ground rules might be implicit or explicit. One of the important ground rules is that arguing, fighting, and emotionally abusive behavior will not be tolerated. I (Ev) prefer to keep this implicit. I try to keep discussions going through me rather than back and forth between partners. I believe that if you let couples fight, except on rare occasions, they will soon conclude that they can fight at home for free. So, they drop out. I (Jen) make the rule explicit if the assessment period appears to indicate this may become a problem, or when I observe it. It's important for couples to understand that the goal of therapy is to learn new ways of relating, and that will be our focus. Old conflictual patterns can be broken, and their underlying needs can still be met in new patterns. Regardless of whether it occurs implicitly or explicitly, the session must feel safe to the couple.

The therapist assigns homework

Homework is vital. Each week is 168 hours. Therapists meet with clients only one "therapy hour" a week. Lasting change requires the couple to try to improve their relationship for more than one "therapy hour" each week. There are two important therapist skills for homework. Therapists must collaborate rather than autocratically assign homework. Then therapists must check at the beginning of the next session on how that homework went. Using therapy time to work through the roadblocks to change at home is key to lasting progress.

Focus on hope

To draw the couple in to their dreams and hopes, the therapist can listen to their origin stories, how their relationships with parents and other romantic partners led to their becoming a couple. The good therapist then can weave a narrative of what they might have hoped and dreamed when they entered this relationship. It could sound something like this:[1]

- "I hear that your childhood was chaotic, and unpredictable. So was your first marriage. When you two moved in together, what hopes did you have for this relationship to be different?" or
- "You enjoyed a happy childhood with loving adults, although you had some struggles, too. When you think back to childhood, what kind of relationship did you dream of?" or
- "I hear fear that the loving, stable, lifetime relationship that you two started is being lost. My guess is that you feel lonely and angry about it. What might happen if therapy works? Can you tell me the ideal story of your future if you could write it?"

The "hopes and dreams" language allows partners to tell their story positively and to feel that the therapist "gets" them. It might have been a long time since partners have expressed their best dreams and hopes to each other. By asking about best dreams and hopes, you subtly communicate that you want them to be happy, not just return to normal semi-misery.

Practical Guidance Through the Assessment

Many people come in contact with your service through initial advertisement, which usually means your website or printed materials that a closely associated health service might provide. You want your website to begin to educate and (if truth be told) start them on the path of healing.

Assessments can be emailed to couples prior to the first meeting or provided through a health app, such as My Chart. Alternatively, and for people not online, questionnaires (see Intervention 9-2) can be provided in hard copy at the first session, and all patients can be instructed to arrive 20 minutes early for that first session.

Intervention 9-2 Pre-meeting Assessment Questionnaires

Whether through your online electronic health record system or old-school paper in the office, questionnaires can help set the baseline, gather information efficiently, and move the couple forward. We have provided a list of assessment instruments we use in Table 9-1. Those we consider most essential are marked with an asterisk.

Table 9-1 Questionnaires and Scales for Clinical Assessment of Couples

General Satisfaction	Couple Assessment of Relationship Elements* (CARE; Worthington et al., 1997); Couple Satisfaction Index (Funk & Rogge, 2007).
Conflict/ Communication	Communication Patterns Questionnaires* (Crenshaw et al., 2017).
Waypower	Relationship Efficacy Measure* (Fincham et al., 2000).
Trust	Dyadic Trust Scale* (Larzelere & Huston, 1980). The Hope project infidelity screening* (hopecouples.com).
Violence	Revised Conflict Tactics Questionnaire* (Straus & Douglas, 2004) or HITS for screening* (Sherin et al., 1998).
Use of Substances	Michigan Alcohol Screening Test* (MAST; Westermeyer et al., 2004); CUDIT-R** for cannabis (Adamson et al, 2010), or Drug Abuse Screening Test** (DAST; Skinner, 1982).
Intimacy	Five intimacy scaling exercise thermometers rating the ideal and current levels of emotional, sexual, social, intellectual, and recreational intimacy. (Two marks on each of five thermometers). A thermometer graphic can be found at hopecouples.com

(*Continued*)

Table 9-1 (Continued)

Problem Identification	What you see as the major problem and two less-severe-yet-important problems you'd like to change in couple counseling* (if you decide to pursue couple therapy). Narrative.
Strengths	Your partner's character strengths: Values in Action Character Test (Seligman et al., 2004); What specific strengths does your partner possess (checklist of 24 virtues).
Forgiveness	Identify an unforgiven hurt that you think might be the most important. (Narrative answer); Injustice gap* (Davis et al., 2015, 4 questions, Emotional Forgiveness Scale* (Worthington et al., 2007, 8 questions), and Decision to Forgive Scale* (Davis et al., 2015, 6 questions) pertaining to that unforgiven hurt.
Religion/ Spirituality (R/S)	What is your religion/spiritual identity?* How prominent is R/S in your lives?* What role (if any) does R/S play in your problems or solutions to your problems?* Did you want to include R/S in your couple therapy?** Essential questions.
Complicating Factors	We have found this list of issues helpful as a checklist*: in-law relationships, gambling, pornography, online/gaming/screen use, eating problems, feelings about my body, sexual behavior that is risky, unwanted attraction to someone of the same sex, pain during intercourse, difficulty with erection, excitement or orgasm, and avoidance of sex.

The dyadic interview typically takes about two hours. We structure it around ten questions that can be written out on a sheet of paper affixed to a clipboard and taken into the interview room to prompt the assessor of the issues to be dealt with. We summarize the ten questions, along with what we are looking for, in each in Intervention 9-3.

Intervention 9-3 The Dyadic Interview Ten Questions

1 **Major problems.** Most people are wound up aching to explain their problems. If you try to redirect the conversation to something more positive without allowing them to do that, they will be frustrated and usually will resist you. So, ask from the beginning, "I'd like to begin by asking you each to tell me briefly what you see as the major problems in your relationship. We'll expand on these as time goes on, but for now, let's just

get a lay of the land." Try to limit how much description you want without making partners feel like you are in a hurry or are cutting them off.

2 **Scaling question.** "Okay, you've told me what you each believe to be the major problems in your relationship. If you had to rate the quality of your relationship *as it stands today* on a scale from 0 = no connection or fully negative connection through 10 = ideal match to my dreams and hopes, where would you see your relationship today?"

3 **Relationship history.** "To help me understand your relationship, would you tell me how you came to meet and then how your attraction grew and how your life together progressed until things started to go sour?" Spend most of the time soliciting information about early attraction and what they liked about each other.

4 **Getting down to specific areas at present.** "It is important that we look at the different areas that make up the relationship as a whole. Many couples come in complaining of difficulty resolving differences. In fact, most people—whether in perfect relationships or very troubled one have at least one topic that they habitually disagree about. I'm going to ask you to discuss one of those issues and record your discussion for seven minutes. (Note: use a HIPAA-compliant device.) I'll look at the recording during the week and be able to know more how we might help you in future discussions. I have a timer that I'll set for 7 minutes. While you are discussing and videoing, I'll be looking at the questionnaires you completed earlier. That will give me a better idea of specific things I can ask you in the rest of our session." When you convene, you can ask them to briefly discuss something they like to do together as a couple. This helps soothe some negative feelings aroused in discussing a topic of disagreement. (You also could have them do that discussion for a second 7-minute recording.) Over the years, we've found it better not leave the couple alone. Hot conflict and even violence can occur. Instead, sit quietly while they discuss. Look over the questionnaires and listen peripherally. Don't make this the last activity of the session. It can leave a lingering negative feeling.

5 **Communication.** You will see them communicate during the video recording, will pick up information through the scales they complete, and will observe them communicate with you. It's helpful to ask them if their discussion with you is similar to how they communicate at home and note differences.

6 **Intimacy.** This is a crucial area to assess because the emotional bond is so important. Many things could disrupt that bond, including sexual

difficulties, emotional negativity due to conflict, and external or family stressors making it difficult to find the time to connect. A frank discussion of sexual intimacy is almost always needed. One time I (Ev) did not conduct such a frank discussion was with a couple about 60 years old. When asked, they smiled and said, "The one area we have always had a good connection is in our sex life. This is pretty much the major reason that we are still together. We are completely satisfied with sex and don't want to change anything about it from how often, to when, to what we do." Okay. I was convinced.

7 **Unforgiven hurts.** Even in the initial assessment, it isn't too early to listen well for (and make a note of) lingering hurts partners are holding onto. Be tentative in such a discussion. We can trigger negative emotions and poison the mood. It's better to hold off a thorough discussion until they have worked on communication, conflict resolution, and intimacy.

8 **Best dreams and hopes.** Since the relationship history, you've been focusing on problems. It's time to turn things around. Open with this. "This gives us a good look at the relationship as it now exists and also how it developed to its present state. But I'd like to end the meeting positively and give you something to think about between now and our next meeting. Then, I'll share feedback with you." Now here's the directive. "Given that you each see problems with the relationship and given that you started the relationship positively and it continued positively until (the event/s, name it), I'd like you each to tell me what you see as your best dreams and hopes for the relationship." Don't rush through this. This is probably one of the best interventions you'll do in this entire assessment session. After they lay out their best dreams and hopes for the relationship, it will help to follow that solution-focused therapy (de Shazer, 1985) directive up with another, the miracle question.

9 **Miracle question.** "If you went to sleep tonight and tomorrow morning, you awakened and your best dreams and hopes had been realized, what would look different in your relationship than happened today?" This will help them be more concrete about what might need to be done to bring about the best dreams and hopes. But it is helpful to take one more solution-focused therapy step.

10 **Moving the needle on your scale.** "Earlier I asked you each to rate the quality of your relationship on a scale from 0 = no connection or fully negative connection through 10 = ideal match to my dreams and hopes. At that time, (one partner's name) rated it 5, and (other partner's name) rated it 6. Can you think of one thing you each could do this week to

move the quality of your relationship just one-half a point higher than you see it right now?" Give each of them the opportunity to come up with something. Then encourage them to do some homework. They can put it on their Couple Improvement Plan worksheet (Figure 9-1)). If you start with homework—and ask about it at the outset of the feedback session—they will likely begin to expect that as a pattern and will fall in with it.

Give Homework at the End of the Intake

One ideal homework for the end of the assessment session is to ask partners to complete Figure 9-1, the Couple Improvement Plan, at home prior to the feedback session (see Intervention 9-4). You must ask about this at the beginning of the feedback session. Therapists who do not follow up on homework they assign soon find that couples won't do the homework.

Intervention 9-4 Assigning Homework and the Couple Improvement Plan Worksheet

"So, you each thought of something you could do in the upcoming week that *might* raise the quality of the relationship by half a point. So, I'd like to ask you to do some homework this week. Are you willing to do a little homework?" (Hopefully, they will agree. If they don't, that, in itself, is diagnostic.) "I'd like you to experiment around and try to raise your rating of the relationship by a half a point. Don't worry about what your partner is doing. You are responsible for trying to raise the quality by what you do, regardless of what your partner does. You just identified something you thought would help, but you might try that out and find it does not really change things. So, keep experimenting until you raise the level."

"I have this Couple Improvement Plan worksheet that helps support couples with this goal. It has several parts to it, and I hope you will use all or most of them each week. It's a place to record your plan for the week. You can have a good time together on a date, as well as a 5-minute 'date' check in on each other's lives most days. There's a place to make plans for self-care and individual goals, as well as to write down gratitude for your partner or relationship. We find getting into the swing of doing this can be tough, especially if you are already pretty discouraged. So, we want to make it easier. On the right, let's decide together right now what is your top 'must do' for the week and identify when you can do these things realistically in your schedule. Later this week, there's a place to write a reflection and to consider what obstacles you are facing that we can discuss and hopefully overcome. We can start simply this week for your goals, but I'm going to ask you to do this worksheet each week. Are you willing to give that a try this week?" Therapists can make their own template, or this one is found at www.hopecouples.com.

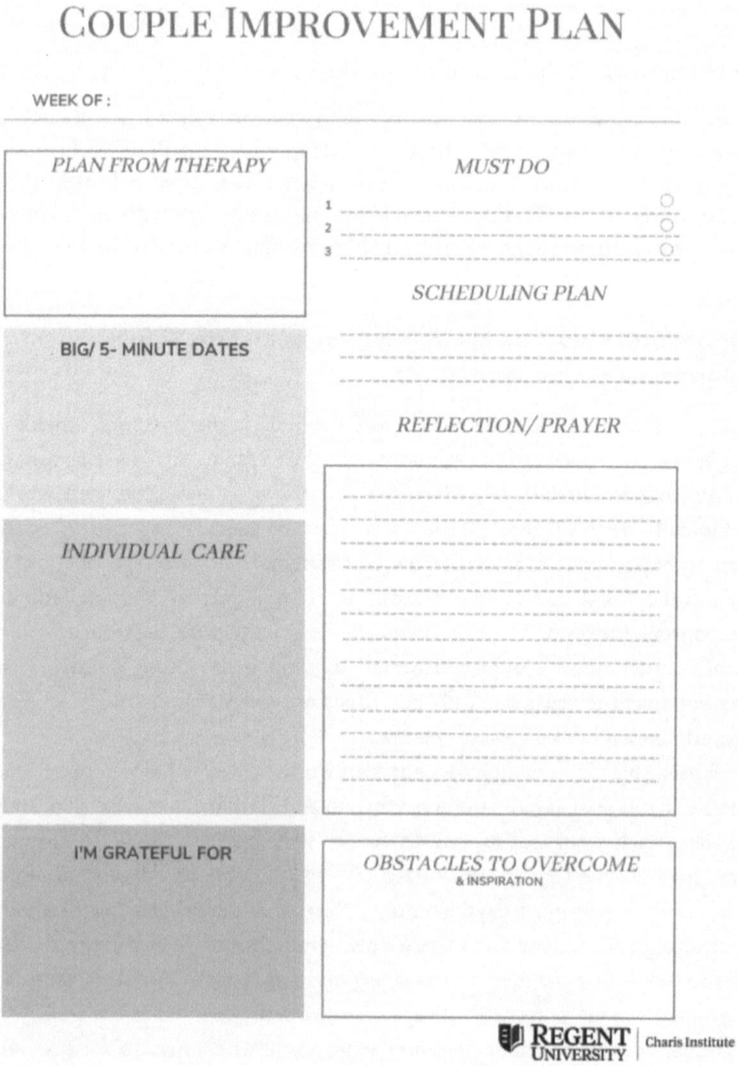
COUPLE IMPROVEMENT PLAN

WEEK OF :

PLAN FROM THERAPY

MUST DO

1

2

3

SCHEDULING PLAN

BIG/ 5- MINUTE DATES

REFLECTION/ PRAYER

INDIVIDUAL CARE

I'M GRATEFUL FOR

OBSTACLES TO OVERCOME
& INSPIRATION

REGENT UNIVERSITY | Charis Institute

Figure 9-1 The Couple Improvement Plan

Red Flags and Individual Intakes

We've all conducted intakes and seen red flags. Red flags are issues that may indicate that couple therapy is contraindicated. There are factors that mark couples as those that almost every therapist would not see for couple therapy: intent on breaking up, substance abuse, domestic violence, infidelity, and untreated significant diagnosis. If these issues arise in your initial questions, then safety is in play. It's important to follow up with details to triage the prescient needs of the couple (see Intervention 9-5).

Intervention 9-5 Detect Red Flags

Think of these in terms of green, yellow, and red flags. No issue. Green flag. Move forward. However, there are often cases with a "yellow flag." Perhaps there is minor substance abuse such as occasional binge drinking, minor domestic violence like rare pushing or pinning without injury, non-sexual infidelities like internet flirting or long-ago history of infidelity. Depression or anxiety are common among people with relationship problems but can complicate treatment. You must assess the level of anxiety or depression and whether it is related primarily to the relationship problems. These "yellow flags" will likely need your attention. Some complicating factors may need focused attention, such as sexual problems that may need a consultation with a medical provider or sex therapist. If a couple has many yellow flags, a therapist should triage with the couple what type of treatment is likely to help them reach their goals best.

Many couples have red flags flying all over the room. But they have become fixated on couple therapy as *the* solution to all their problems. It feels like a major car accident has arrived in the office and the patient insists that acupuncture will fix everything. But it seems clear that surgery is needed. Red flags indicate meaningful problems. We are here to handle problems, so it's important not to shame couple or make them feel like you don't want to help them. Couples with red flags are often the most fragile and discouraged, having adjusted to pathology for years. Our job is to help the red-flag person access specialized care. A referral to a psychologist well-versed in forensic care, severe mental illness, or substance abuse may be needed.

It's a waste of everyone's time to do regular couple therapy and ignore red flags, or even many waving yellow flags. In fact, in the case of red flags, you can actually harm partners by ignoring problems. The issues around the problems will need significant attention and, generally, some individual therapy may be needed before or simultaneous with couple therapy.

Should we have individual intakes? Individual intakes are especially important if you have yellow or red flags. If in doubt, it's best to indicate that individual intakes are normal and schedule your next meetings individually. Sometimes, individual intakes are just to follow up on a few issues of potential psychopathology or questions about things that you couldn't get to in your dyadic interview timeframe. Other times, you have real concerns about whether their relational needs might be secondary to substance abuse, violence, or other red flags.

How long are individual intakes? Will you need half or full sessions? You must ensure you have all the information you need to launch into feedback and treatment plan without missing key information. However, you also have your couple at the highest level of motivation for change at your first meeting with them, so capitalizing on that motivation to see quick change is important. You don't want to spend weeks between initial contact and feedback. It's a balance.

Conclusion

In this chapter, we have helped you get started. In detail. Perhaps more detail than you wanted. Many couples terminate couple therapy after a very few sessions. We believe that much attention up front to pre-therapy preparation, assessment, and intake will reduce those premature dropouts—and research supports this belief.

Note

1 Credit to Jim Sells PhD for his way of phrasing these hopes and dreams intake questions.

References

Adamson, S. J., Kay-Lambkin, F. J., Baker, A. L., Lewin, T. J., Thornton, L., Kelly, B. J., & Sellman, J. D. (2010). An improved brief measure of cannabis misuse: The Cannabis Use Disorders Identification Test – Revised (CUDIT-R). *Drug and Alcohol Dependence 110,* 137–143.

Crenshaw, A. O., Christensen, A., Baucom, D. H., Epstein, N. B., & Baucom, B. R. W. (2017). Revised scoring and improved reliability for the Communication Patterns Questionnaire. *Psychological Assessment, 29*(7), 913–925. https://doi.org/10.1037/pas0000385

Davis, D. E., Hook, J. N., Van Tongeren, D. R., DeBlaere, C., Rice, K. G., & Worthington, E. L., Jr. (2015). Making a decision to forgive. *Journal of Counseling Psychology, 62*, 280–288. https://doi.org/10.1037/cou0000054

de Shazer, S (1985). *Keys to Solution in Brief Therapy*. W. W. Norton.

Fincham, F. D., Harold, G., & Gano-Phillips, S. (2000). The longitudinal relation between attributions and marital satisfaction: Direction of effects and role of efficacy expectations. *Journal of Family Psychology, 14*, 267–285.
Fisher, R., Ury, W. L., & Patton. B. (2011). *Getting to Yes: Negotiating Agreement Without Giving In*. Penguin Books.
Friedman, E. H. (2017). *A Failure of Nerve: Leadership in the Age of the Quick Fix*. Church Publishing.
Funk, J. L., & Rogge, R. D. (2007). Testing the ruler with item response theory: Increasing precision of measurement for relationship satisfaction with the Couples Satisfaction Index. *Journal of Family Psychology, 21*(4), 572–583. https://doi.org/10.1037/0893-3200.21.4.572
Howard, K. I., Lueger, R. J., Maling, M. S., & Martinovich, Z. (1993). A phase model of psychotherapy outcome: Causal mediation of change. *Journal of Consulting and Clinical Psychology, 61*(4), 678–685. https://doi.org/10.1037//oo22-006x.61.4.678
Larzelere, R. E., & Huston, T. L. (1980). The Dyadic Trust Scale: Toward understanding interpersonal trust in close relationships. *Journal of Marriage and Family, 42*, 595–604.
Seligman, M. E. P., Park, N., & Peterson, C. (2004). The Values in Action (VIA) classification of character strengths. Ricerche di Psicologia, 27(1), 63–78.
Sherin, K. M., Sinacore, J. M., Xiao-Qiang, L., Zitter, R. E., & Shakil, A., (1998). HITS: A short domestic violence screening tool for use in a family practice. *Clinical Research and Methods, 30*, 508–512.
Skinner, H. A. (1982). The Drug Abuse Screening Test. *Addictive Behavior, 7*(4), 363–371.
Swift, J. K., Callahan, J. L., & Vollmer, B. M. (2011). Preferences. In J. C. Norcross (Ed.), Psychotherapy Relationships that Work: Evidence-Based Responsiveness (pp. 301–315). Oxford University Press.
Swift, J. K., & Greenberg, R. P. (2012). Premature discontinuation in adult psychotherapy: A meta-analysis. *Journal of Consulting and Clinical Psychology, 80*(4), 547–559. https://doilorg/10.1037/a0028226
Swift, J. K., & Greenberg, R. P. (2014a). *Premature Termination in Psychotherapy: Strategies for Engaging Clients and Improving Outcomes*. APA Books.
Swift, J. K., & Greenberg, R. P. (2014b). A treatment by disorder meta-analysis of dropout from psychotherapy. *Journal of Psychotherapy Integration, 24*(3), 193–207. https://doi.org/10.1037/a0037512
Swift, J. K., Penix, E. A., & Li, A. (2023). A meta-analysis of the effects of role induction in psychotherapy. Psychotherapy, 60(3), 342–354. https://doi.org/10.1037/pst0000475
Straus, M. A., & Douglas, E. M. (2004). A Short Form of the Revised Conflict Tactics Scales, and Typologies for Severity and Mutuality. *Violence and Victims, 19*(5), 507–520. https://doi.org/10.1891/vivi.19.5.507.63686
Westermeyer, J., Yargic, I., & Thuras, P. (2004). Michigan Assessment-Screening Test for Alcohol and Drugs (MAST/AD): Evaluation in a Clinical Sample. *American Journal on Addictions, 13*(2), 151–162. https://doi.org/10.1080/10550490490435948
Worthington, E. L., Jr. (1989). *Marriage Counseling: A Christian Approach to Counseling Couples*. Downers Grove, IL: InterVarsity Press.
Worthington, E. L., Jr., Hight, T. L., Ripley, J. S., Perrone, K. M., Kurusu, T. A., & Jones, D. R. (1997). Strategic hope-focused relationship-enrichment counseling with individual couples. *Journal of Counseling Psychology, 44*, 381–389.

Worthington, E. L., Jr., Hook, J., Utsey, S., Williams, J., & Neil, R. (2007). *Decisional and emotional forgiveness*. Paper presented at the International Positive Psychology Summit, Washington, DC, Oct 5, 2007.
Worthington, E. L., Jr., McCullough, M. E., Shortz, J. L., Mindes, E. J., Sandage, S. J., & Chartrand, J. M. (1995). Can marital assessment and feedback improve marriages? Assessment as a brief marital enrichment procedure. *Journal of Counseling Psychology, 42*, 466–475.

10 Providing Feedback to the Couple

Engage Couples in Planning Their Treatment

Problem: How to provide feedback that will be sticky?
Solution: Create clear written feedback with specific plans.

If you have ever sat in the client's seat in a therapist's office, you know the feeling of wondering what your therapist really thinks. Some of that may be our own insecurities, but it is extremely difficult in the early stage of therapy for a therapist to communicate all the issues and perspectives. Yet, the therapist's perspective is a major reason why therapy helps clients! Couples need access to your thoughts as their therapist. Many approaches to couple therapy spend an entire session explaining the theory of change and therapist's perspective. However, we know that verbal communication alone has poor retention, while written communication can clarify and strengthen retention. We think that a written report with verbal discussion is the best way to give this feedback.

After the intake, hope-focused therapists write an assessment report. Both partners get a copy. That report shows your commitment to engaging with and helping the couple. Its positive (though realistic) tone help build trust and faith in therapy, if undertaken, and in your ability to work with couples in general and with them in particular. The centerpiece of the feedback is the assessment report, which contains the facts of the relationship and your evaluation.

Starting the Feedback Session

How you start the feedback session is crucial. After you've greeted them, inquire about how their week went. If they complain, empathize but don't get sucked into trying to fix their problems, do therapy, or even give advice. Your contract with them was assessment and feedback.

DOI: 10.4324/9781003009382-12

If things went well, often the couple will talk about their efforts to raise the quality of the relationship by half a point. If they don't raise that spontaneously, you *must* ask. If you do not ask and do not deal with it seriously when they bring it up, then couple therapy will likely never benefit by homework. Because they probably won't do it.

If they did not succeed with raising the relationship quality by half a point, treat that as diagnostic. You can observe, "I'm sorry you had difficulty with that homework. Assigning homework and observing how you handled it was part of the assessment. I'm encouraged that you each tried to make the relationship better. I'm sorry that you couldn't succeed."

After discussing the homework, ask the partners to reflect on what they felt after last week's assessments. Allow them to express themselves. That can lead to discussing the assessment report. Hand a copy to each partner and tell them you'll email another copy after the session. Allow them to read the whole report. Then, discuss it section by section.

The construction of the report is standardized even though its content will be couple-specific. Its standardization makes it easy to write in less than an hour. In Intervention 10-1, we provide guidance in the make-up of the report. Because it's helpful to actually see an example, in Intervention 10-2, we show one. Note how the structure will always be the same.

Intervention 10-1 The Assessment Report

The assessment report is a great alliance builder. It shows that the therapist assessed carefully and respected the couple enough to listen and get the details of the relationship correct. It also shows that the therapist is willing to spend time to create the report. The report looks as if it might have taken hours to prepare, but an experienced therapist can create a template that describes what most couples share—things like high conflict, disrupted communication, more negative than positive interactions, loss of hope, erosion of faith in each other and in the relationship, little effort being put into bettering the relationship, and loss of love shown by treating each other poorly and not actively valuing each other.

The report begins with the vital statistics of the partners and a statement of each's major complaints. Importantly, it then reports the partners' major hopes and dreams for the relationship within the next four months. Place these before relationship history to highlight what the couple are shooting to accomplish.

Next comes a summary of the relationship history, which moves the facts of the relationship to the present. Even though we don't skimp on positives early in the history, partners can become discouraged because their relationship is troubled now. Good questionnaires, notes (or video review), and careful listening will populate your report with information. The sections on personal data and presenting complaints are exercises in paying attention to what the partners said in the assessment session. Unless we made errors of fact (which undermine couples' confidence), partners usually have little to say in those sections.

We follow that with an assay of their strengths. Try to find some strengths that relate to faith, work, and love. Your assay of weaknesses also groups by faith, work, and love. Recommended goals for treatment use those same categories to suggest targets for treatment. Suggested treatment goals are tentative because, as discussion takes place, things might change.

We include an overall evaluative paragraph, which is aimed at evaluating the needs partners and relationship. At the end of the report, we make a clear recommendation about therapy. If we recommend therapy, we provide a separate tentative, session-by-session treatment plan.

Intervention 10-2 Feedback Report Example

CONFIDENTIAL

Carl and Sarah Simpson (Fictitious Names)

Personal Data

Carl (37) and Sarah (36), married for seven years, have sought counseling because they want to improve their marriage, which has recently had more frequent conflict and less intimacy. They have three children: Michael (6), Paul (5), and Esther (2). Paul has recently been diagnosed with an attention deficit disorder with hyperactivity (ADDH) by the educational psychologist in their school district. Carl reports a close relationship with his mother, who lives nearby. Sarah reports estrangement from her parents, who live in Illinois and are divorced.

Presenting Complaints

Carl and Sarah feel discouraged by their marriage. They argue often over many topics—notably tensions about the amount of work-related time that

Carl spends at work and home, sexual relations (frequency), child-rearing concerns around Paul's ADDH, and different religious involvement. Both feel unappreciated and devalued—especially during conflict but extending into many areas of the relationship. They feel that they must attend counseling to give it a try, but they wonder if counseling will help.

Hopes and Dreams

Carl and Sarah at first had trouble identifying their hopes and dreams for the marriage. But after some thought and discussion, they both agreed that they wanted to stop arguing, not just to be silent but to agree more and talk about differences without getting angry. They also both wanted to rekindle earlier feelings of love for each other. Carl hopes for affection and a strong sexual bond. Sarah hopes to feel that they support each other in co-parenting their children and are better friends.

Relationship History

Carl and Sarah met nine years ago. Carl was line supervisor and Sarah was a worker on the line. Sarah initiated the contact, and they began seeing each other. They had seen each other for two years at marriage.

They conceived on their honeymoon in Jamaica. Michael was born at the beginning of their tenth month of marriage. Neither felt ready for parenthood. Carl felt increasing pressure to support the family financially. He began to spend more time at work. With Paul's birth, both parents felt an increase in demands on their time. Carl sold his Corvette and entered a local community college. He received degrees and earned a promotion. But the recent graduation has started new arguments.

Relationship Strengths

The relationship is strengthened by having two caring partners, both of whom are very interested in making the marriage work. When asked about their partner's top traits, Sarah said Carl is steadfast, a never-give-up attitude, and fun-loving. Carl said that Sarah is usually attentive to his emotional needs, spiritually mature, and funny. Their high commitment to each other and to working at counseling is a sign of personal strengths that have carried them this far and will help them reach their goals.

Relationship Weaknesses

Three weaknesses plague the marriage.

- Love for each other is weak. Pressure and conflict have intensified differences, and both Carl and Sarah feel devalued for what they do or who they are.
- The relationship has been neglected. It needs work. Like a garden that needs weeding, marital weeds are choking out the fruit of love. They have gotten used to being disconnected.
- The relationship is short on faith. Both partners have lost faith in their own ability to solve marriage problems. Both have little faith that counseling will help their marriage. In fact, this struggle with faith at all levels is highly distressing to both partners who usually see themselves as faithful people.

Recommended Treatment Goals (or Goals to Work Toward Even if Couple Therapy Is Not Entered)

Hopes and dreams for the marriage. When asked how they would know if their marriage was better, Carl and Sarah agreed that the marriage would be better if they went through a weekend without any arguments (Carl's idea) or made love and cuddled afterward (Sarah's idea). Let's keep these in mind.

What is needed to improve the relationship? Improvement happens through bettering love, work, and faith.

- **Love** is being willing to value and refusing to devalue each other.
- **Work** is putting energy into maintaining and improving your relationship.
- **Faith** is trusting in each other and in your ability to resolve differences with mutual satisfaction.

How can these be bettered?

- They said they would like to **value** each other more by showing more explicit appreciation for each other. Valuing could also include making more effort to do things that they know their partner wants. For one example each: Carl could pick up clothes more often, and Sarah could stop reminding Carl of what he needs to do as often.

- **Work** (aka spend time) on the marriage with humility and perseverance. Concentrate on the next six months while the marriage is repairing itself.
- Have **faith** that their work on the marriage will pay off. Try to observe positive changes with an open mind and try to call attention to positive changes they observe.

Measurement. They were asked to scale their satisfaction from 0 = none to 10 = perfect. They agreed it was 3 most days. They indicated that they are dissatisfied in most areas. Their highest rating was commitment; their lowest, communication.

Baseline Couple Satisfaction Index

Carl: Dissatisfied. 3/10
Sarah: Dissatisfied. 3/10

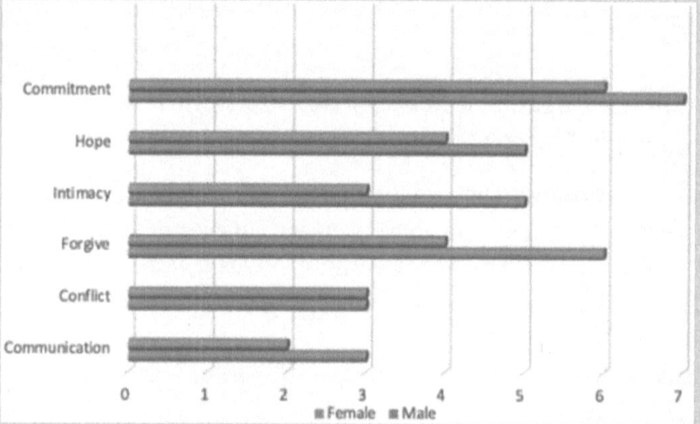

They were each asked, "What could you do tomorrow to bless your partner enough to raise your own and your partner's satisfaction by 0.5." Carl said he could pick up his clothes and hug Sarah affectionately (not sexually) three times that day. Sarah said that she could not make critical statements all day and tell Carl three different things she loved about him. Both thought that if they carried out those actions, that would make a big change. They agreed to try those prior to this feedback report, and if those actions didn't help, find something else that might.

Overall Summary

Carl and Sarah's marriage is troubled by conflict and low intimacy, but they have a good foundation. They love each other and share many common values. They are committed to the marriage and the family. Their problems can be resolved, and love restored, **if Carl and Sarah are willing to work hard on their relationship**. The changes in their relationship depend largely on how hard they are willing to work and on whether they are able and willing to love each other by valuing each other. They are encouraged to draw on their faith in the relationship to help them **work with high energy on it**.

Recommendation

Based on this overall assessment, I believe that Carl and Sarah would benefit by 15 sessions of couple therapy. Our agreement was to undergo this assessment and feedback and then discuss options for improving the relationship. I have prepared a tentative treatment plan for us to discuss. We can also talk about other options.

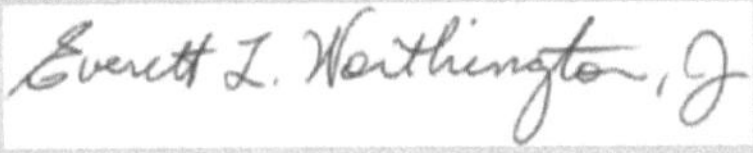

/Signed Everett L. Worthington Jr., Ph.D./

Designing an Overall Treatment Plan

The plan

Our students—and even practicing professionals—always want more on how to design a strategic treatment plan. Below, we describe how to use the strategy of promoting love, work, and faith in constructing a plan.

Length of treatment

Ultimate success depends on accurately estimating duration of treatment. We can't predict external stressors or resistances that might slow down progress. So, we use ongoing assessment of where the couple are, where they want to be, and obstacles that can interfere to stay responsive to the couple. But accurately estimating the optimal length of therapy is the first step.

Treatment involves work

Recall that most couples don't believe therapy will take more than a few weeks. Armed with lots of research, we know better. Begin with the idea that they need to commit to at least 40 hours of working on their relationship. (Provide information about research on typical durations of treatment.)

Make a clear recommendation about length of treatment

It is better to over-estimate the duration needed than to under-estimate. Some couples treat the recommendation as a contract. If they are not fully better at the recommended duration, they might end anyway. That usually spells relapse. Few couples ever get upset if you and they think they are done 12 sessions through an 18-session recommended treatment.

Provide the four-step plan

Most treatment involves three stages—building hope through relationship skills early in treatment, building intimacy bonds directly in the mid-stage of treatment, and repairing damaged bonds in the final stage. Then, that is followed by termination that solidifies changes. Thus, the treatment plan is structured in these four sections. Couples differ in how many sessions they have in different sections.

Remember, interventions are only a means to the end of modifying the emotional bond so that problems are mitigated and good functioning is likely. Select interventions based on your experience and the couple's preferences. Interventions are not magic. Here are some principles we use to decide which interventions to recommend in the treatment plan:

- High-conflict couples need time-out interventions first to stop a conflict cycle with a better interaction. Use interventions with high structure and direction.
- Disengaged couples who are living parallel lives with little interaction need indirect bond building. Use bonding skills and forgiveness.
- Highly conscientious or perfectionistic couples need relaxed de-pressurized relationship time. Encourage them to slow down and enjoy each other.
- Partners who are low in self-esteem benefit by positive interventions, like gratitude or appreciation.
- Almost all couples benefit from talking calmly, productively, and with care about their real concerns. Many exercises can help with that goal.
- Entrenched couples need exercises that break up patterns. Genograms can help hopeless couples gain hope; critical and defensive couples develop a new narrative as to why they struggle.
- In the mid-phase, use interventions that help partners emotionally connect. If you read a technique in this book and think, *That might make them cry*, then consider it for mid-treatment.

- Many couples can't easily identify one specific hurt to focus on forgiveness. Their hurts are too numerous. Yet, almost all couples struggle with lack of forgiveness. Help couples identify an exemplar hurt each partner experienced. Work through forgiving and repairing the relationship using confession and amends making. This is typically best done after working on communication and conflict resolution.
- Termination is not necessarily a one-and-done final good-bye session. Process learning in therapy, solidify gains, and open the door for follow-up or re-engagement with therapy if needed. Clearly, termination will be more complicated if the couple attends 26 sessions than if they attend 8 sessions.

With these guiding principles and specific suggestions in mind, let's look at an example treatment plan for Carl and Sarah (see Intervention 10-3).

Intervention 10-3 Example Treatment Plan for Couple Therapy

Potential Treatment Plan if Carl and Sarah Enter Couple Therapy

I recommend couple therapy for 15 sessions within the next 18 weeks.

The Work: In the assessment, we identified the need for hard work on the marriage. Sarah and Carl, we ask that you focus *one work week* (**about 40 hours**) of effort on your relationship while attending therapy. That "work week" will include 15 hours of therapy and 25 hours of positive "homework" together working to improve your relationship. That averages about 2 hours a week.

When people come to therapy, most expect that they will need only about 4 sessions to set things right. This is rarely the case. Fewer than 20 percent will be successful in 4 sessions of therapy. To set realistic expectations, let me tell you the research. Research has found this.

> Between 13 and 18 sessions are needed for 50 percent of patients to feel good about ending therapy. Between 20 and 26 sessions are associated with about 80 percent of patients successfully ending therapy.
>
> If you are like most people, based on an 18-week duration, there are three phases of therapy. In the first, you'll increase hope for 2 to 4 sessions. But often a dip in hope follows, because all problems are not quickly resolved within four weeks and a brief setback is normal. In the second

phase, by around session 12, symptoms usually have decreased. It is easy to think therapy is done, but usually that is a false assumption. In the third phase, from sessions 13 to 18, lasting change is practiced and becomes more habitual. Ending treatment before functionality is re-established—even though symptoms might have decreased by then—can bring a relapse of symptoms.

Here is my suggested tentative plan for what we might address. This is subject to your (Sarah and Carl's) input and, of course, might be adjusted depending on circumstances.

Week 1–5: Communication and Conflict-Resolution Skill-Building

Week 1: Reducing and Managing Conflict (observing your conflict; the difference between positions and interests; negative reciprocity). Use of time-out disengagement when needed.

Week 2: Resolving Differences without Conflict (listen and repeat; observe your effects; leveling and editing); review by using the LOVE acronym.

Week 3: Reducing and Managing Conflict (Harvard Negotiating Project—Getting to Yes; identifying underlying interests).

Week 4: Communication of Positive Affect (PAR), Gratitude, and the Love Bank.

Week 5: TANGO-E, combining good communication with underlying interests. Prepare for genogram intervention next week.

Week 6–8: Bond Building

Week 6: Family Genogram, reflecting on patterns of closeness and tension in family history, and your relationship history.

Week 7: Increase sexual intimacy through dates and play.

Week 8: Create more elaborate shared hopes and dreams for the relationship.

Week 9–12 Addressing Hurts from the Past and Preparing for Future Repairs

Week 9: Forgiveness—learn REACH forgiveness; homework = complete the 2.5-hour DIY-workbook on REACH forgiveness.

Week 10: Ask questions about forgiveness raised by workbook; tackle hard-to-forgive hurts.

Week 11: Reconciliation Four Steps; assess where you are; plan to move to the next level.

Week 12: Read letters of forgiveness; discuss use of apology and forgiveness in future hurts; check-in on progress; consider whether ready for reconciliation.

Week 13–15 Turning Toward the Future

(You can space out these meetings if it fits schedules.)

Week 13: Lingering concerns; reconsider hopes and dreams and the degree to which they have been realized; if not, plan for reaching or revising them; grace and acceptance of self and partner as humans with enduring weaknesses.

Week 14: Discuss gains made in couple therapy; plan for temporary relapses and crises and decide how to deal with them; homework = create a "graduation" project together.

Week 15: Re-evaluation; either extend and arrive at a treatment plan for those sessions, or (hopefully) terminate and plan for solidifying gains and moving forward.

If couple therapy is not desired, then this treatment plan can provide ideas of ways that might be employed at home for you to improve their relationship. Resources are available without cost at www.hopecouples.com and www.EvWorthington-forgiveness.com.

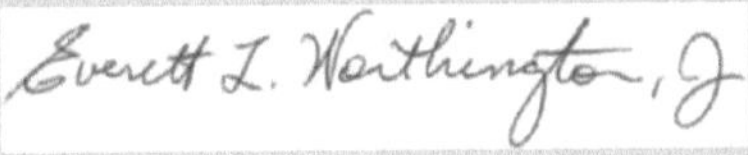

/Signed Everett L. Worthington Jr., Ph.D./

Negotiating the Treatment

In the end, the duration of treatment and what happens during treatment are the couple's decisions. But you must give your expert opinion and recommendation and explain your thinking behind those. It is usually not a good idea to undertake a treatment plan that is substantially less than you believe is necessary for success. However, that said, often we agree to something less if you can also agree that periodic reassessments will inform whether modifications need to be made to the plan.

It is necessary to use routine outcome monitoring to keep informing treatment throughout its conduct. But, in cases where there are wide differences between your and the couple's estimate of what amount of therapy is needed, routine outcome monitoring becomes crucial. To that, we turn our attention in the next chapter.

Conclusion

Feedback is not giving a personalized psychoeducational lecture to the couple. Feedback is not the meaningless ratings we give after a visit to our local pharmacy, intended to make us feel listened to. Feedback is a collaborative, patient-responsive conversation using our prepared report as a way of co-constructing a treatment plan with the couple that they will feel co-ownership for.

11 Setting Up Routine Outcome Monitoring

Put Assessment to Work

Problem: The client's voice needs to be clearly heard and issues addressed.
Solution: Routine outcome monitoring gives clients a clear voice and place to reflect on their growth

Long gone are the days when we counseled couples for 15 weeks and trusted that, because they looked okay and wanted to terminate, we could assume that couple therapy was a success. We now know that such an approach pales in effectiveness to what we do now.

Routine Outcome Monitoring (ROM)

ROM keeps both our own and the couple's fingers on the pulse of the relationship. ROM's power is to engage everyone in a discussion of what is and isn't working. It also invites open conversation about hard to address topics like resistance and allows quick repair of ruptures in therapeutic bonds throughout treatment (see Intervention 11-1).

Intervention 11-1 Routine Outcome Monitoring (ROM) Assessment

Ask the couple to complete the ROM at the beginning of the session each week. For in-person clients, make the form available on paper when they check in. For online clients, use an email link to an online questionnaire with their appointment reminder. We also create a welcome message with a link

DOI: 10.4324/9781003009382-13

or QR code in the digital waiting room, which increases last-minute participation. Address any reluctance or skipping this activity. That might indicate deeper issues of demoralization about the relationship or therapy. Process low or unexpected scores immediately at the beginning of the session.

Research shows that ROM increases the efficacy of treatment (Tilden & Wampold, 2017) by increasing couple satisfaction, decreasing dropouts, and allowing problems to be discussed soon after they occur. It gives voice to clients who might otherwise hold back on issues like, "I really hoped we would talk about sex, but we don't" or "I feel like the therapist is on my partner's side, not mine." ROM also implies to couples that we expect change, and they are the pivotal part of making it happen. It is consistent with patient-responsive treatment, which is assumed nowadays by most couples.

ROM is tailored to our approach

ROM works best when it fits with the therapy approach. If existing ROM systems fit your approach, you could employ them. Examples are the Partners for Change Outcome Monitoring System (PCOMS; Sparks & Duncan, 2018), Outcome Questionnaire-45 (OQ-45; Burlingame et al., 1996), or the Systemic Therapy Inventory of Change (STIC; Pinsof, 2017). We have developed the Hope-ROM approach, which ties directly to concepts in the hope-focused couple approach (HFCA) model. We include it in Figure 11-1 and invite you to use it.

There are three sections. Four questions (rated 1 to 5 each; total 20 points) concern the relationship. Two questions (rated 1–10; total 20 points) concern the therapeutic relationship. One question (rated 1–20; total 20 points) concerns individual well-being of the partner completing the H-ROM. This 20-point per target structure provides a picture in which you can track progress on the same graph.

Therapeutic application of ROM weekly

It is important to take the time in counseling to look at the results of the weekly survey.

- If they indicate a concern, address immediately.
- If both partners report that they are improving, encourage and praise their hard work.

HOPE ROUTINE OUTCOME MONITORING

PERSONAL INFORMATION:

NAME: ______________________ DATE: __________

COMPLETING THIS ○ Before session ○ After session

INSTRUCTIONS:

Answer each question about how you feel about your relationship THIS WEEK

QUESTIONS:	RATING SCALE:				
	Never 1	Rarely 2	Sometimes 3	Often 4	Always 5
Emotional Engagement: Do you feel you are emotionally connected, (trusting, open, safe) with your partner this week?	○	○	○	○	○
Understand: Do you feel you understand and are in tune with each other?	○	○	○	○	○
Alliance. Do you feel like you and your partner are working well together toward relationship goals?	○	○	○	○	○
Work. Are you putting time and effort into improving your relationship (doing positive/ healthy things for your relationship)?	○	○	○	○	○
	Never 1	Rarely 3	Sometimes 5	Often 8	Always 10
Therapist alliance. How much is your therapist working with you to accomplish your goals?	○	○	○	○	○
Would you say Couple Counseling is working? We are working on the things I want to work on in couple counseling.	○	○	○	○	○

	Couldn't be worse 1									Couldn't be better 20
Overall, what is your level of well-being (how you are doing)?	○	○	○	○	○	○	○	○	○	○

Did you use any exercises, resources or recommendations from couple therapy this week? If so, how did it go?	

Figure 11-1 H-ROM Questionnaire

- If the partners see things differently, explore why. It is not unusual for one partner to perceive the relationship to be more positive than the other partner. Common reasons include possible power struggles between partners, projecting past interpersonal patterns with parents or other authorities (e.g., medical caregivers or teachers), personality differences, or one person experiencing psychological symptoms.
- If they plateau, which is common after the remoralization phase, try to discern why. Ask what they think. They might have experienced a rise in hope during early sessions and think, this is good enough, so they let their effort wane. If the partners indicate that they continue to be dissatisfied with their relationship with the therapist or if they feel that their emotional bond is perennially troubled, have a conversation about those.
- Pay attention to the therapy relationship ratings. In our experience, couples rate therapy more highly in general than they rate their relationship bond. So, pay close attention if therapy ratings drop. Even moderate ratings of therapy would warrant slowing down and processing how their needs are not being met. The therapist might ask questions like "What is causing the gap for each of you between what you are experiencing in therapy and what you would like to see?"
- What if they have low scores? Very low scores on the relationship rating require special attention. It's often not helpful to reveal the low score directly; that can demoralize and spark an in-session flood of emotions. An open conversation is often better than a graphic. When a therapist sees a drop in the rating, or a stubborn low score, it is very important to ask open questions about the needs of each partner to determine the meaning. Partners who are unwilling to discuss their needs with their partner, but report low scores on the form, have a problem that will stymie the progress of treatment. They may need specific help asking for what they need directly but kindly. If partners continue to have low scores after 7–8 sessions of couple therapy, then an open and frank conversation about whether something can change for the better or whether they want to consider another approach—like a different treatment plan or reassessment for psychopathology.

Periodic check-in

Every 2 or 3 weeks, therapists should present these results for discussion as a computerized line chart (like Excel), or hand-drawn (something like Figure 11-2). There would be a chart for each partner to review. In the chart, you can include the 3 components—relationship bond, satisfaction with therapy, and individual well-being. We have left off the therapeutic relationship line in our example because it seemed to confuse couples to

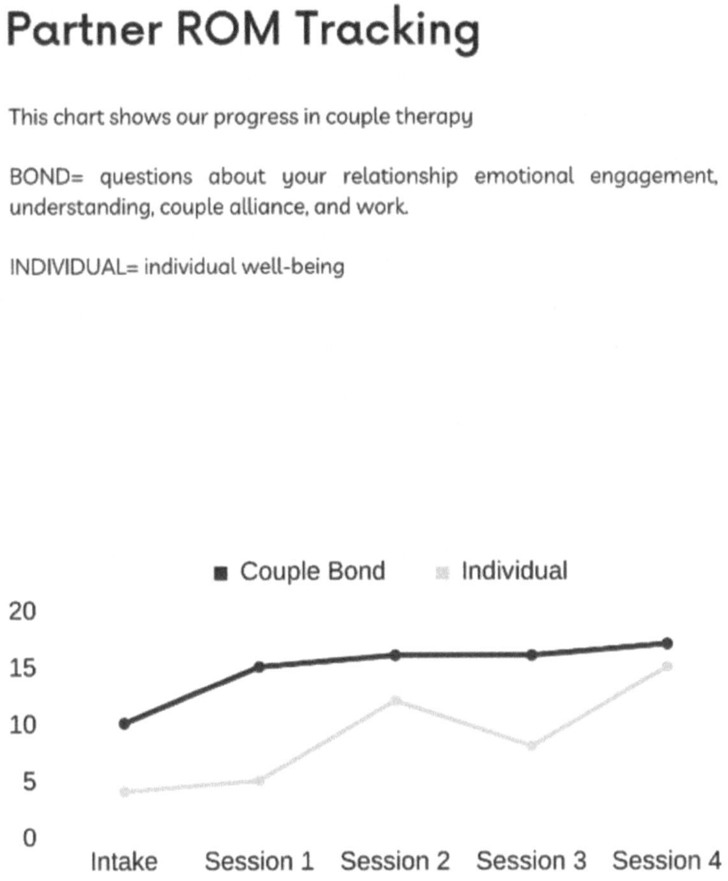

Figure 11-2 Line chart tracking scores of weekly ROMs

have 3 lines, and typically the therapeutic relationship score is very high throughout treatment.

Conclusion

We have spent a lot of time talking you through the initial assessment, feedback, and ROM. We think that, while ROM is not considered to be "owned" by couple therapy, it is a foundation from which couple therapy (and each session) launches. Therefore, it is a crucial aspect of couple therapy. These three chapters have outlined steps to therapy that give it a structure for change. This beginning creates a warm and welcoming on-ramp to therapy, clearly informs the couple about what HFCA offers, emphasizes homework as well as in-session interventions, invites collaboration, and sets up the expectation that progress needs to be watched often. Now we are ready to consider the interventions that are within HOPE.

References

Burlingame, G. M., Umphress, V., Hansen, N. B., Vermeersh, D. A., Clouse, G. C. & Yanchar, S. C. (1996). The reliability and validity of the Outcome Questionnaire. *Clinical Psychology and Psychotherapy, 3,* 249–258.

Pinsof, W. M. (2017). The Systemic Therapy Inventory of Change—STIC: A multi-systemic and multi-dimensional system to integrate science into psychotherapeutic practice. In T. Tilden & B. E. Wampold (Eds.), *Routine Outcome Monitoring in Couple and Family Therapy: The Empirically Informed Therapist* (pp. 85–101). Springer International Publishing. https://doi.org/10.1007/978-3-319-50675-3_5

Sparks J. A., & Duncan, B. L. (2018). The partners for change outcome management system: A both/and system for collaborative practice. *Family Process, 57,* 800–816.

Tilden, T., & Wampold, B. E. (Eds.). (2017). *Routine Outcome Monitoring in Couple and Family Therapy: The Empirically Informed Therapist.* Springer International Publishing.

12 Using Couple Therapy Methods for Hope

Instill Hope for the Holy, Hurting, and Healthy

Problem:	Instilling hope in couples.
Solution:	A good strategy and techniques will increase hope.

One main goal of couple therapy is to instill enough hope that the couple will sustain indefinite work to improve and maintain their relationship. It's like watching a home improvement show.

Hope for a Better Home

You watch the beautiful home emerge, and you look around your own living room, and say, "Ya know, I think I could improve that wall there." You start to order the materials to improve your own home. The show gave you hope and the means to better your wall. Good relationship improvement and maintenance have to be done at regular intervals: keeping pesky critical attitudes at bay, fixing small hurts before they become large, and creating beautiful experiences that bond partners.

When we watch home improvement shows, there is a theme of healthy, hurting, or holy. Some rooms are perfectly *healthy* spaces. We think, *That room's not too shabby. In fact, it looks better than this room.* But suddenly the space is even more beautiful. It inspires us to reach for health and beauty. In some makeover shows, the target is a *hurting* house stuck in 1965. At the end, it's a completely new space. It takes extensive work, but the outcome is jaw-dropping. Many families shed tears at that level of improvements. But there's one more type of hope—for the *holy*. This is the miraculous extreme makeover with hosts like Ty Pennington. A family is on the brink of ruin, stressed to the max. The home is saved from demolition or bankruptcy by the show. The children get to go to college. The family is no longer considering homelessness. The show plays the role of angel or Jedi knight ("Help us, Obi-wan Kenobi, you're our only hope.")

DOI: 10.4324/9781003009382-14

How do you instill hope for health, hurting, or holy needs? We rely on the techniques (more specifics to come in future chapters on that) implemented with a strategy of faith, work, and love. It's not that couples don't know *how* to relate well to each other. If we offered them a million dollars to relate well for one day, you can bet they would be kind and loving. It's the same as home dilapidation. Slow neglect or catastrophic processes have caused people to say, "What's the use in trying? I could work hard for days and not see much change." Partners may think they would have to work for improvement alone while their partner continues to cause damage. Couple therapy is all about home improvement: Equipping two people with creative ideas to make things beautiful, motivating them until hope becomes self-sustaining.

While all of the techniques of the hope-focused couple approach (HFCA) can produce hope, we offer two ideas here to get hope ball rolling. These illuminate patterns that are often misunderstood or full of blame, withdrawal, and contempt.

Illumination of Their Communication Patterns

The first task is to help partners become aware of how they are relating to each other. On one level, they are very aware that they are not behaving as they ought. On another level, few are aware of how they contribute to the cyclical patterns. To help get a more objective view of their own behavior, we suggest a video review (see Intervention 12-1).

Intervention 12-1 The Video Review

When a couple is really stuck, struggling, and throwing all their best blocking resistances to change, we have found the video review can unstick them. It can break up the pattern of a therapist working hard to get the couple to change while they resist. Other couple therapy approaches use this same intervention (e.g., Gottman), so there seems to be a convergence that this is often effective.

The process is simple. Couples make a video recording. Remember that HIPAA-compliant video recording is important if you do it. Or have the couple record on their own phones. Just like the intake, the couple creates a video re-enacting an argument. Or they can agree to record in the midst of an argument during a session.

The therapist can say, "Let's create a recording of this communication and see what can be learned. I will record for you for 7 minutes. You all discuss this as best you can." Record and set it up for replay.

Ask the couple to watch themselves for how they could have done anything better. The therapist can rewind the tape to a spot where each partner can see where things might have gone better. After the replay, ask each of them what they noticed. It's uncanny how many couples get tearful as they watch themselves just 10 minutes earlier, angry and anxious.

To close this intervention, encourage partners to write 1–3 basic ideas from the intervention in a journal or their couple improvement plan worksheet. There is great power in watching the video and writing lessons learned.

Video review allows for a powerful "third-person perspective" on communication. The third person is the impartial video "eye." It's important not to let the couple use the recording as a tool to bash their partner. Rather, keep them focused on what they could have done better—not their partner. Focusing on how to improve communication uses positive psychology principles, which are more motivational in the long term than calling out the partner's negativity.

Breaking Up Negative Patterns

Another technique used across many theories, mostly behavioral and cognitive-behavioral, is stopping negative reciprocity. This is responding to some action or communication perceived to be negative with a reciprocal negative action. The negative emotion ramps up quickly to explosive levels. Negative reciprocity can explain quick reactive conflict or even hostile and aggressive interactions (Cordova et al., 1993). Perceived hostility is often met with more hostile actions.

Conditions like brain injury, extreme stress, trauma, feelings of helplessness, or a general proclivity toward violence set the stage for negative reciprocity. But frankly, it can happen to anyone. Anger is a common reaction to anger.

The purposes of Intervention 12-2 are to (1) illuminate negative reciprocity cycles and (2) create strategies for stopping them. This intervention is aimed at being able to practice emotional regulation, positive communication, and conflict resolution. Changing negative reciprocity can be framed as a courageous, generous, or gracious response to a stressful situation.

Intervention 12-2 Stopping Negative Reciprocity

Therapist and couple explore how negative reciprocity works. Get partners' views about whether it occurs and, if so, how often. If it fits to use distancer–pursuer patterns (Guerin et al., 1996) as the foundation of the intervention, that can work well. Portray the enemy as the destructive *pattern of negative reciprocity* when partners seek to self-protect instead of collaborate.

Solicit suggestions about how partners might eliminate negative reciprocity. Some couples may need to have this intervention coupled with time out, self-care, emotional regulation, or self-soothing interventions.

Tell the couple that the real trick is for them to practice and use their ideas in the heat of the moment. Use role-play or attempt simple behavioral rehearsal during a session. Most couples in therapy will have difficulty stopping a negative reciprocity cycle without much practice. Knowledge is not usually enough. The less emotionally regulated the partners, the more support will be needed.

An alternative version of this model labels the cycle as pain–defense–offense (Sells & Yarhouse, 2011; adapted in Figure 12-1). Discuss how a partner experiences pain, inside or outside of the relationship. The partner attempts to defend themselves from that pain as a normal human response. However, that defense is often offensive to their partner. For example, a partner might withdraw by reading a book to defend against

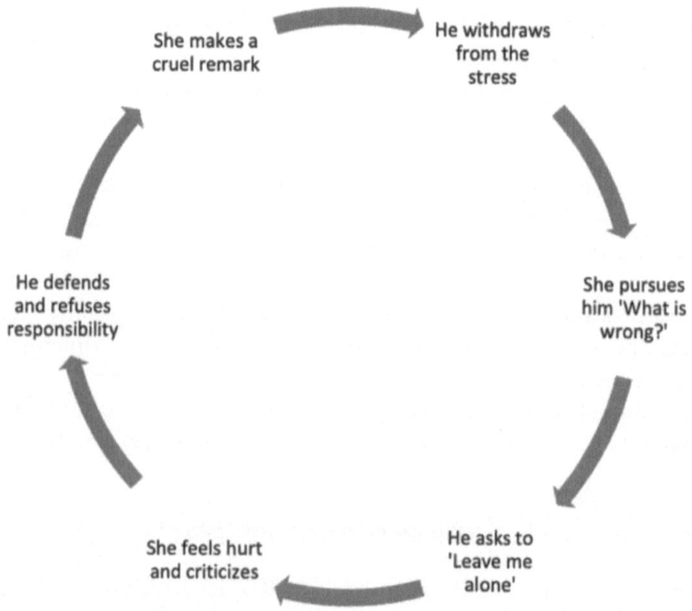
She makes a cruel remark
He withdraws from the stress
She pursues him 'What is wrong?'
He asks to 'Leave me alone'
She feels hurt and criticizes
He defends and refuses responsibility

Figure 12-1 Pain–Defense–Offense Pattern (adapted from Sells & Yarhouse, 2011)

negative emotions, but their partner feels ignored, which is offensive. Almost every couple can use real-world examples of a pain–defense–offense pattern to illuminate their cycle, which increases hope for change, sustaining the work of therapy.

Conclusion

As we move toward the intervention-heavy portion of the book, we begin by covering two communication interventions that are used often across different theories. In the next chapter, we'll move on to discuss conflict resolution.

References

Cordova, J. V., Jacobson, N. S., Gottman, J. M., Rushe, R., & Cox, G. (1993). Negative reciprocity and communication in couples with a violent husband. *Journal of Abnormal Psychology (1965)*, *102*(4), 559–564. https://doi.org/10.1037/0021-843X.102.4.559

Guerin, P. J., Jr., Fogarty, T. F., Fay, L. F., & Kautto, J. G. (1996). *Working with relationship triangles: One-two-three of psychotherapy*. Guilford Press.

Sells, J. N., & Yarhouse, M. A. (2011). *Counseling Couples in Conflict: A Relational Restoration Model*. IVP Academic.

13 Helping Resolve Conflicts

Find Mutual Interests Beneath Surface Fights

Problem: Conflicts are painful.
Solution: Identify the couple conflict cascade and intervene with powerful techniques.

Any family or roommate can tell you that conflict comes with the package of living in near proximity to someone. This is even more so with couples, who share identity, resources, and living space and need each other for goals such as companionship, financial savings, and sex. The conflicts are noxious to the couple, therapists, their family, and anyone else who witnesses the breakdown.

Why Does Conflict Happen?

Why we fight instead of hug

Why do people push away the person they *say* they want to be most close and loving? Furthermore, the partners can be paragons of sensitivity, empathy, and generosity all day long. Then, at night they might be at each other's throats. Surely character ought to overcome their conflict. But it doesn't.

Why? Perhaps you remember the dual-processing model of the brain popularized by Daniel Kahneman (2011)? Fast and slow pathways of the brain create the potential for reactivity in close relationships. Slow rational thinking governs what we ought to do. Fast thinking is reactive. Reactivity goes up when people are distracted, stressed, under demand, and leaning into rehearsed communication patterns. Couples tend to be together in the most tired, distracted, yet demanding parts of their day, after they have expended much of their concentration or physical labor at work.

DOI: 10.4324/9781003009382-15

Weeknights from 6pm to bedtime and weekends are packed with activities, meal-making, exercise, kids' activities, home maintenance, errands, elder care, religious or social meetings, and *maybe* a little time to escape into a show, savor a good book, or fool around. The few hours a week the couple might be able to interact as friends, lovers, co-parents, or in groups of people are too few and often pressurized. And that assumes the couple is not facing health or mental health challenges or external stressors. Bottom line—reactivity is expected!

Worse. The more it's practiced, the more it's expected. Repeated reactivity can easily lead to a "default mode" of threat detection in the brain (Gronchi & Giovanelli, 2018). Threat detection is deeply ingrained in the human mind, even when we are safe, we are always looking for a threat. Also, patterns just get stamped in with practice.

Couples pay us to help them get better but they spend all week reacting harshly to each other, assuming the relationship is hopeless and their partner doesn't love them. This is not a skill-deficit problem fixed by the perfect conflict-management education. This is an alligator problem. Alligators are well-adapted to survival. They grab now, ask questions later. Conflict is usually deep in the fast emotion pathways of the brain where attachments lie. And by the time couples get to therapy, it is almost always a deep fast-thinking, reactive problem.

How fighting moves the couple toward dissolution

John Gottman's theory (1993, 2011) is a schematic of how relationship distress leads toward dissolution. The negative cascade is based on research with thousands of couples. There is a balance of positivity versus negativity in all relationships. At inflection points, couples either turn towards each other or away from each other. When the emotional balance is too negative, partners move away from each other.

This is like a cascade in a river. It starts small at the beginning. If water is not absorbed or rerouted, the flow keeps growing. If not stopped, flooding results.

When couples turn toward each other, the destructive waters are diverted to more productive uses. When couples turn away from each other often enough, waters build a splashing, dashing cascade that the Gottman calls, the four horsemen of the apocalypse (i.e., criticism, defensiveness, contempt, and stonewalling/war) which are traditional harbingers of the end-times.

This leads to unfavorable attitudes and attributions. Once this happens the bond begins to erode in the relationship. This creates the Zeigarnik effect, which is that unfinished or unprocessed conflict has much more power than processed conflict. Continually turning away from each other feeds the cascade because you cannot process issues. Unprocessed conflict is like a waterfall, speeding the flood forward. If such conflict-floods happen often enough, the couple falls further into distancing, avoiding conflict, having secrets, betraying, not trusting, and finally recreating a negative history. In the end, couples often say, "I don't think we ever really loved each other. I never should have trusted this person." If a couple in therapy is late in the process, then addressing their history to row back against the current will be needed.

Dam it

Instead of letting the negative floods flow, couples must make dam-like moves. We do this by encouraging couples to turn towards each other more often, to stop the four horsemen at criticism if possible, and to examine attributions about the relationship. By resolving issues, we defeat the Zeiganik effect, not leaving unprocessed issues hanging to garner power. This doesn't mean couples far down the cascade can't recover. But it's more difficult for them. It will be like an extreme home makeover and require more time and energy.

Apply work, faith, and love to reverse the cascade

In the hope-focused couple approach (HFCA), we use the cascade model of conflict to help couples resolve conflicts. (Thank you Dr. Gottman.) First, we help couples observe what is going on when they have conflict. Help them discern whether they are in chronic criticism, defensiveness, contempt, or either stonewalling or war. This will take work, require rebuilding faith and trust, and challenge partners to value each other and not devalue each other. We offer below many techniques and interventions that we have found effective in our clinics. In Figure 13-1, we have summarized the major aspects of the process of couple conflict, leading to intervention.

Turn-Towards-the-Partner Interventions

LOVE

LOVE is one of the most highly rated interventions in our practice (see Intervention 13-1). Just before COVID-19 broke out in early 2020, Ev and his wife, Kirby, were at a community play. At intermission, the couple sitting behind them tapped Ev on the shoulder. "You're Dr. Worthington, right?" asked the man. Ev fessed up. "We were in your study in 1999 on

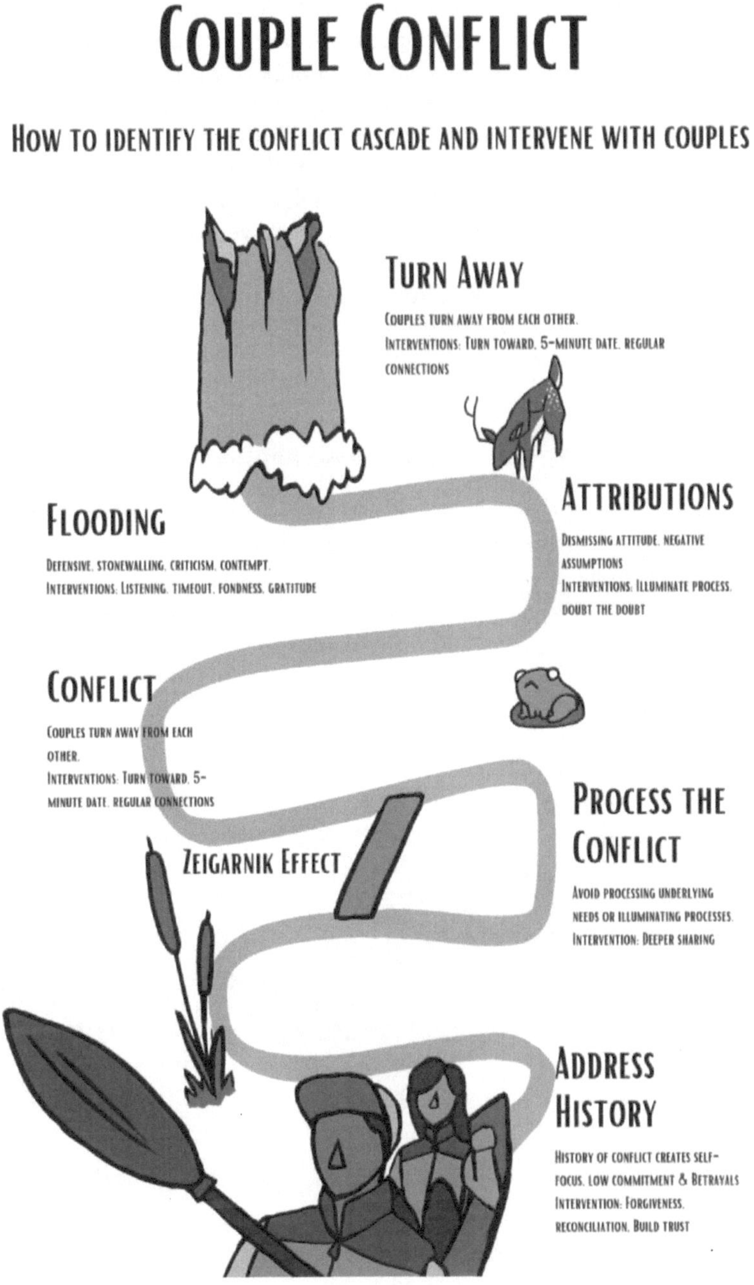

Figure 13-1 Couple Conflict: Process and Intervention

early married couples. We learned the HOPE intervention that gave us an assessment of our marriage and then taught us about communication, conflict negotiation, and intimacy. That nine hours of counseling did wonders for our marriage. When the study started, we had been married only six months. We were having many arguments. We were drawn to the project hoping to smooth out some of those problems. Your couple therapist taught us the LOVE interventions. That pretty much eliminated our fussing."

"Look at us, now" the wife chimed in. "We've been married 21 years, we are at a play together, still holding hands. And when we do argue, we usually can get past it quickly. And," she continued, "we laminated the paper with the LOVE acronym on it. It's still attached to our refrigerator! We even taught it to our teen daughters."

Intervention 13-1 LOVE—Three Interventions in One

This intervention is especially helpful earlier in the process to help couples turn towards each other, or to help with processing a past conflict. The LOVE acrostic is actually three interventions plus a reminder always to value and not devalue the partner, even in the midst of a heated negotiation about differences (see Figure 13-2).

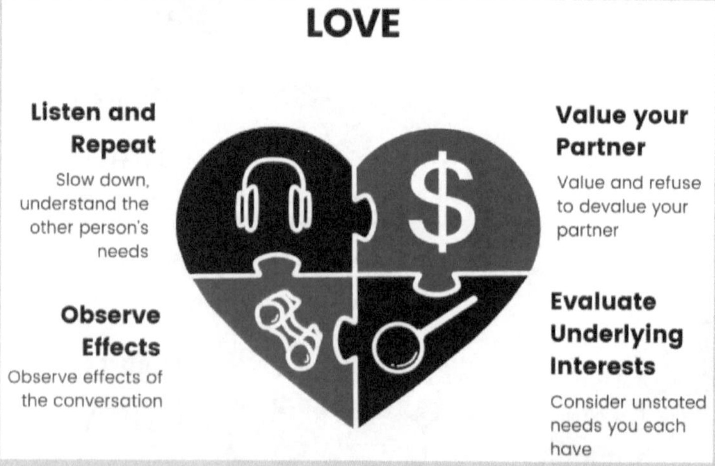

Figure 13-2 The LOVE Acronym

L stands for listen and repeat, which is a way of breaking up both partners' competition to be understood by stopping and trying to ensure that they have understood the partner. It is familiar to every mental health professional because we encounter it in our listening-skills training.

O is to observe one's effects. The cue to tune in to what effect the speaker is having is when the partner does not act according to expectation. The speaker should stop and ask why. If conflict continues, perhaps call a time-out and enter into a cool-down contract.

V is to engage the principle of valuing your partner.

E is to evaluate the interests behind one's position in a conflict (Fisher et al., 2011). This is the Harvard Negotiation Project method. Common interests often hide behind incompatible positions. Partners learn to sense when they seem to be at an impasse and consider what they really want, that their position might be obscuring, and ask the partner also to identify interests behind their position. Often a win–win solution will emerge. We'll take this up in detail in Intervention 13-8.

Make time for connection

The five-minute-date intervention (see Intervention 13-2) helps couples connect in everyday ways. In the midst of conflict, couples often withdraw or avoid each other, even on simple things like shared chores or co-parenting.

Intervention 13–2 Five-Minute Date

The five-minute date encourages couples to set aside five minutes each day to check on each other's lives. Ask how work was. Connect about the friend they are worried about. See how the kids' event was.

Couples in frequent conflict often need to schedule this. Some couples seem to attempt to avoid even this simple connection—which is diagnostic. Re-establishing normative cooperation and checking in on each other is key to getting partners to turn towards each other.

Four-Horsemen Interventions

Listen and repeat (see Intervention 13-3; this was also L in LOVE, Intervention 13-1)

When the four horsemen have descended on the field, very simple interventions are needed. Some couples have the capacity to simply stop arguing or trying to make their point and instead say "OK, you talk. I will listen.

I may not agree with you but take your time and tell me what you are thinking." If they have the ability to do this naturally at home without therapist intervention, you are in a good place to send the four horsemen packing. Those willing and able to try this in their next argument often get the positive experience of a much better outcome than a jousting event of conflict. If couples can hold hands, or have warm touch during their listening activity research indicates they will have better physiological reactivity than those who don't hand-hold (Conradi et al., 2020).

Intervention 13-3 Simple Listen and Repeat, Warmly

This is probably only going to work with couples whose conflict has not yet become chronic. There are two parts.

1 Partners agree to use listen and repeat. Decide who will listen first.
2 Coach partners in active listening rather than passive listening that does not respond to what the talker is saying.

Practice the TANGO

The TANGO and TANGO-E are typically used as exercises in listening. They will be explained in the following chapter (Intervention 14-6) and so we mention them just to alert you that they are possible ways to break up toxic conflict also. Couples rate these highest in our lab in data collected over the last 20 years.

Time-out from hot conflicts

Time-out is an emotional anti-flooding intervention, like a levee on a dam that holds back the flood waters from further damage (see Intervention 13-4). When the flood waters overtake us, no one is going to be boating. The best choice is to take a rest, and let the flood waters come down. Research indicates that the ability to stop negative, emotion-driven, dysfunctional, and destructive interpersonal activity is an important central goal of all couple interventions (Bradbury & Bodenmann, 2020).

Intervention 13-4 Time-Out

Help couples learn to "conflict observe." Work with them to notice the signs when they, or their partner, are getting flooded with negative emotions. When they can accept that nothing good is likely to happen, either partner can call a time-out. Set a time, relatively soon, to resume the discussion. Now. Coach partners that the time-out is simply to let emotion recede, not time to think up the winning argument. Give ideas for how to spend the time-out in healthy activities like exercise, watching a show, playing a video game, or reading.

Several problems can arise when attempting to use time-out with distancer–pursuer couples (Guerin et al., 1996). The first is that pursuers struggle with stopping the conflict. They may need behavioral rehearsal in self-soothing and distraction when emotionally triggered. The second is that distancers don't want to resume the discussion. They may need self-soothing techniques to calm fears of re-engagement.

Expressing love

One antidote to criticism and contempt in particular is expressing valuing love and admiration for one's partner (see Intervention 13-5; this was also V in Intervention 13-1). Ideally, partners can put in sincere statements of love even as they are expressing their differences. That may not be possible during a strong conflict for some people. They might need to build up a reservoir of love that can be drawn on in times of conflict.

Intervention 13–5 Expressing Valuing Love

Let partners know that it is important not to lose sight of mutual feelings of love even when heatedly disagreeing. Suggest that there are two frequent conditions.

1 Reassure your partner that you still love them even though right now you are disagreeing. Coach partners that they can say things like, "I'm really upset right now, but I want you to be reassured that, even though we are disagreeing, I still love you."
2 Build up a bank of love when things are going smoothly. Start by determining how you each like to be shown love. One way to do that is using Chapman's (1996) best-selling book to determine each partner's favorite love languages. Then practice showing love in ways that are appreciated. That will go a long way to keep emotions under some control during disagreements.

Express gratitude to keep conflict in perspective

Gratitude can sometimes keep the four horsemen at bay. Gratitude is being thankful or appreciative of something. There is some (but not much) research that gratitude is associated with well-maintained relationships (Gordon et al., 2012). Partners who felt appreciated and valued, tended to show more appreciation, be more committed, cooperative, and positive in their relationship. Theoretically, all of these effects are thought to increase the bond between partners.

This might suggest that couple therapists can use gratitude interventions to help repair damage done by arguing. There is little direct research to support gratitude as a relationship intervention. There is much general research on brief gratitude interventions with individuals, like keeping a gratitude journal. Davis et al. (2016) meta-analyzed studies of brief gratitude interventions. With tongue firmly in cheek, they entitled their article, "Thankful for Little Things" because effects were weak but consistent. Gratitude helps, but it won't turn around troubled relationships *on its own*. Gratitude interventions might be useful in keeping conflict in perspective (see Intervention 13-6).

Intervention 13-6 Experiencing and Expressing Gratitude

Partners who have had a conflict might be approached something like this. "I know you are both feeling angry after that discussion (argument). I'm going to ask you to do something really difficult. Something you probably won't like at first. But this might help you put the discussion (argument) in a wider context. I'd like you each to say whether you'd be willing to come up with some things you are sincerely grateful for about your partner. It's tempting when you've just had a heated discussion (argument) to be a little passive-aggressive in doing this, but I'd like you to consider whether you can be sincere."

1 Solicit whether they each are willing.
2 Ask one partner to name several things they are grateful for in the partner.
3 Ask the other.

Conclude by saying, "I know this doesn't change your feelings about the discussion. But I hope it shows that you are working toward restoring a relationship that you value with a person that you value."

In my (Jen's) own practice, when I have the highest conflict couples in the office, I have employed gratitude interventions. Gratitude is not the only antidote to conflict, but it's accessible for discouraged partners and can spark hope that change can happen. It can be used as part of the Couple Improvement Plan worksheet. Gratitude does not require one's partner to do anything. It can be done as part of homework and journaling during times of lower conflict in the day. Most partners who are not at the highest level of hostility and conflict want to turn things around. Gratitude is generally accepted as an individually healthy activity, so even if the partner is on the fence about leaving the relationship, engaging in gratitude for the partner and the relationship has value. Reading gratitude lists in the next meeting also helps the meeting start in a soft, cooperative framework.

Interventions to Shift Attributions

Attributions are private beliefs about what is causing something to happen. Negative attributions can cause a brief flare-up to become an oft-voiced reason to break up.

A couple once arrived in session and reported that the guy had brought home flowers for his wife, and she had proceeded to ask him, "what did you do now?" This negative attribution for a positive event was an opportunity for illumination of patterns for the couple. His intentions were being doubted. This intervention allows you to work with the couple as a team to identify in which situations they might make negative attributions about ambiguous, neutral, positive, or negative behaviors. Intervention 13-7 aims to help couples question or doubt their negative attributions (doubts).

Intervention 13-7 Doubt your Doubt

We all make attributions of cause about our relationship or about the partner. Therapists can help partners understand how their attributions for their partner's behaviors are an important step in conflicts. Negative attributions can lead to increased anger, detachment, or conflict.

Give examples. We might think, he forgot my birthday because he's passive-aggressive or she is negative all the time because she hates me; he forgot my birthday because he's under a lot of stress, or she is negative because she's been depressed for the last month.

Notice that some attributions of cause are unchangeable—like being passive-aggressive as a personality trait or hating the partner as a stable emotional stance. But other attributions of cause are more temporary—like being under stress or experiencing depression. Actually, few things are truly unchangeable, but we often treat our attributions as if the cause is unchangeable.

Invite partners to examine their own attributions, especially the negative ones, and see if they are attributing cause to things they don't believe can be changed.

If partners find unchangeable negative attributions, ask them to see whether they think they might do something unexpected that might make the attribution more positive.

Give examples. If a private attribution was, she is negative because she hates me, then could the person check this out by asking her, or could he find times when she was not negative or times when she showed love instead of hate.

Conclude this. If you are doubting your partner, perhaps it is because of your own attribution. If you can check this out (by doubting your own doubt), you might find that your attribution needs to be replaced by a different one.

Conflict Interventions

Diffusing a power struggle

One couple seen in therapy reported that sex was good for the first twenty years of marriage, but between ages 45 and 50, the wife went through menopause and began to feel pain during intercourse due to less lubrication of her vagina. She pulled back from sex from once weekly, to something closer to once monthly. The husband's prostate specific antigen began to climb and he was diagnosed by his urologist as having an enlarged prostate (but no sign of cancer). This led to some erectile challenges, which even medication could not completely solve. He was still really interested in sex. Their discussions were not characterized by problem solving. They were in a power struggle.

In therapy, they laid out the problems on both sides. Then the partners turned to the therapist. The wife said, "What should we do? We are feeling our love life slip away, and we want to recapture it." The husband chimed in, "Just tell us what to do and we'll do it."

With an invitation like that, it is tempting for the therapist to think, *Perhaps I can come up with a suggestion in which I offer a balanced solution, with both husband and wife "giving" equally.* This is a trap that the wary therapist does not want to fall for. The issue is not solving the problem although that seems the goal on the surface. The issue is who can say how things are going to play out—in a word, power.

One way to approach this is to use the Getting-to-Yes method in Intervention 13-8 (this is also E in Intervention 13-1). But perhaps you might need to give it a slight twist.

Intervention 13-8 Diffusing a Power Struggle by Setting up a Win–Win and Inviting Partners to Honor Each Other's Valued Choices[1]

The Harvard Negotiation Project method is, in a nutshell, simple. It helps people avoid locking into mutually exclusive "positions" and instead identifies each person's interests behind the position they advocate. The idea is that compromises force each side to give up some part of what they want. If mutual interests can be found, a win–win solution may be possible.

Yes, sounds simple. In practice, the positions are already targets for power that are heavily invested. Also, most couples don't think in terms of "interests" behind their positions. Even translating this into "deep down, what would you really like to have happen?" rarely clears up communication. You can imagine the couple with the power struggle over sex saying, "I'd really like to have sex more" and "I'd really not like to have sex as much." Not helpful. We find that, when "interests"-talk fails, it can be helpful to fall back on talking about the "values behind what you'd like to have happen."

The with-a-twist conversation might go like this. The therapist might say, "You each seem to have suffered physical changes that disrupted your previously satisfying sex life. It seems that you'd like to recapture that. But, because this has gone on for quite a while, this probably will not be as simple as finding a compromise. You have both thought deeply about possible solutions. None have worked so far."

The therapist dodges the gold-gilded invitation to provide a compromise solution, which both partners would likely shoot down. Instead, the therapist invites them to talk about what is important to them. So, the therapist invites an exploration of the underlying values and why they are valued so much. Finally, the therapist suggests that the partners honor each other's valued choices and be willing to give on less important issues. In a ninja therapist move, the goal is to get the couple to move away from arguing about the best solution and dialogue about their values and goals. You can set them up for success by suggesting that they honor each other's highest value or goal.

Sorting out important values

A popular intervention in the Hope couple counseling lab is the values card sort (see Intervention 13-9). This is useful with less verbal and less introspective partners, with younger couples, and with couples pursuing enrichment rather than therapy. It generates a discussion of values.

Intervention 13-9 Values Card Sort

The couple identifies 10+ values in session or as homework. Couples can generate their own values or the therapist can offer a list of values and their definitions that couples can select from or supplement. We have used this list, and we include their definitions. Acceptance, extended-family relationships, parenting, romance, social contacts, tranquility, honor, social status, order, power, fairness, independence, idealism, pleasure, basic needs, security, saving for the future, spiritual transcendence, sexual enjoyment, emotional support, personal growth, family traditions, fun activities, and hobbies.

Type values on cards and give each partner a set.

They create three lists: Essential, Important, and Less-important values, then they discuss their lists. Have partners take a picture of their card sorts to remember for the future.

Interventions to Process Conflicts

Process conflicts realistically

Partners are helped to talk calmly about how and why a conflict went badly. They seek to understand the partner's perspective. They might also repair the relationship damage by apologies and forgiveness. Perhaps they might learn how to avoid similar problems in the future.

When discussing conflict, a big mistake is that each partner repeatedly tries prove they were right and also enlist the therapist on their side. Getting them to process the conflict (see Intervention 13-10) undercuts implicit assumptions and fantasies that the partner will give in. The goal is a deeper level of sharing than they have been doing as they argue their point.

Intervention 13-10 Process the Conflict

Start with this analogy. "If we shove regrettable incidents under the rug, it gets lumpy and we can trip over the lumps. We need to lift the corner and sweep out the old dirt and let it go."

- Instruct them to assume that each will have a different view—both correct, just different.
- Say that an apology (for the sake of merely moving on) is meaningless unless one understands what the apology is for. An apology is not just saying you're sorry for what you did. It acknowledges that you understand why the partner felt hurt.
- Find out what each person did, thinks the partner did, and how it affects the relationship.
- Ask each person to take responsibility for what they did and for the hurtful impact on the partner, even if they didn't intend it to have that impact.
- Urge partners to put their desire to win behind what is good for the relationship and for the partner.
- If it is felt, each partner can express remorse and apologize (i.e., vulnerability).

Repair damage done during conflict

In conflict, masters of relationships can repair the damage done. Everyone gets cranky and negative at times and conflicts happen. Masters of relationships, however, can step back after they calm down and say something like, "I'm sorry. That did not come out like I intended it to. Can we try this again?"

The basis of being able to repair and regulate conflict is friendship. Friends understand and are fond of each other. They turn toward each other for emotional connection, and they can repair conflict damage. Once again, we are indebted to the Gottmans' research and clinical expertise (Gottman & Gottman, 2015). Discussing past conflicts and attempting to repair them will require a soft start-up (see Intervention 13–11), which signals open engagement, friendship, fondness, and appreciation when starting a difficult conversation.

Intervention 13-11 Begin Hard Discussions with a Soft Start-Up

Describe (a) the necessity of a soft start-up and (b) the benefits of setting the tone of discussion and in keeping emotions moderated. (c) Give contrasting examples—a harsh versus soft start-up. Then (d) have partners try starting a touchy conversation softly.

Here are two contrasting examples. A husband did many chores around the house this week besides those he usually did. His husband seemed to take them for granted. A harsh start-up might be to say, "I'm pissed. I busted my tail all week doing extra things around the house, but you didn't seem to notice. You should be more observant and sensitive. You seem self-absorbed and seem like you don't appreciate me."

A soft start-up might be, "I'm upset. I know you've been under stress at work, and I've been there myself. I appreciate you aren't coming home and dumping that stress on me. I know that such pressures can really focus us internally. I've tried to take the pressure off of you by doing extra chores this week, like (names three chores). I would feel better if you acknowledged what I've done because I care for you."

The slimy pit

This intervention (see Intervention 13-12) is inspired by Steven Hayes's (Praxis CET, 2023) Drop-the-Rope exercise. Hayes applies this to individuals in psychotherapy. We have adapted it for couples. The goal is to help partners detach (or de-fuse) from the unwanted impact of emotions, thoughts, or ideas. This detaching is also known as defusion. The intervention uses a physical metaphor. Each of our interventions, you'll recall, aims at making change sensible, that is, able to be sensed in ways in addition to talking and listening.

Intervention 13-12 Slimy Pit Demonstration

The purpose of this intervention is to demonstrate that wrestling with individual emotional negativity or relationship negativity will pull them into a pit of unending pain and will prevent them from pursuing positive dreams and goals.

- Ask partners to identify painful interpersonal "monsters" in their emotions and thoughts. These might be individual, such as, "No one will ever truly love me because I am a failure." Or they may pertain to the relationship, such as, "Why try, I will fail at this relationship too." The painful monsters demand time and attention. They will suck us into an emotional pit that pulls us away from a good relationship.
- Have partners note what things in their relationship they long for or hope for, such as peaceful enjoyment of their relationship or a sense of growth and accomplishment.

- Ask partners to stand up. Get their agreement to participate in a demonstration.
- Tell them their hopes and dreams are located across the room, out of reach, but the painful monsters are in a slimy pit right in front of them.
- Pick up a rope. Ask one partner to hold the end of the rope. Say that you are going to pull each of them into the slimy pit of monster pain while their partner sits quietly and doesn't help.
- Ask if they would like to resist being dragged into the pit.
- Begin to pull gently and gradually increase your force. Let them tug back on the rope. After they have pulled a while, note that they have done well to resist. Also note that fighting negativity is tiring.
- Ask, what would they like to do now? Many will want to involve the partner. The partner might help tug on the rope for a while.
- Eventually, or sometimes soon, most people realize they want to drop the rope and stop the struggle. When they ask permission, you can say, "My job is to pull you into the pit. You have to decide how to prevent that." Many will drop the rope.
- Pick up the end and offer it to them again, saying, "Good!" Often, they will take the rope back. Start pulling again.
- Offer the rope several times while you are talking with them about something else. Say, "Here just hold onto this for a minute." Slowly begin to pull them toward the pit again.
- Have them identify power struggles or gridlocked chronic arguments they engage in as a couple. Then identify relationship values, dreams, and goals, they are not pursuing when they engage in the struggle. Some examples are connection, enjoyment, peace, and pleasure. Have them really reflect on what they long for, what they really miss, and what they hope for. Then, have them take the rope and pull hard on the rope with each other to demonstrate power struggles between them. After they have struggled, ask whether they want to drop the rope here as well.
- The point, of course, is that if they keep picking up and fighting the rope, their goals and values will not be enjoyed. They need to support each other, drop the rope, and walk across the room to their values, dreams, and hopes.
- Sit again. Process what they experienced. Was it easy to get sucked back into picking up the rope? The main learning is to experience the way struggle makes you want to "win." So, it can be self-perpetuating

Conclusion

Duong (2023) studied 775 students from three universities who completed a course on intellectual humility. We end this chapter by summarizing the five lessons below. You'll see a remarkable convergence with the methods discussed in this chapter.

1 **Let go of winning.** Don't approach a potentially divisive conversation like a zero-sum game. That activates competition. It sets up one person to fail. Instead, enter conversations with intellectual humility and curiosity. Try to understand the other person, which can breed reciprocity.
2 **Share your story and invite others to do the same.** People rarely change their minds about deeply held beliefs because of facts. You might open new doors by sharing stories about your own experiences. Discuss issues through your experience of them. Tell why you find an issue to be important. Invite the other person to share their personal experiences. Try to draw out common insights.
3 **Ask honest questions to understand.** Instead of manipulative or gotcha-type questions, ask nonjudgmental questions that invite reflection.
4 **Acknowledge the role of emotions.** Try to validate the other person's feelings about an issue. You can do that without agreeing with their beliefs. By acknowledging their feelings, you say that you hear them, which can foster trust. They might even become more open to your view.
5 **When possible, seek common ground.** Common ground can be found in shared goals, interests, or values. Connections based on common ground are tools that build relationships, which can lead to other points of connection.

Helping partners resolve conflicts is not merely promoting intellectual humility. Relationships have dynamics that can drive even the most intellectually humble duo to impasses. But if we had to advise couples of individual character dispositions to foster, intellectual humility would be right up there with love, empathy, general humility, and forgivingness.

Note

1 Drawn from *Getting to Yes* by Fisher, Ury, and Patton (2011) and also from the Gottman Method Couples Therapy by J. M. Gottman & J. S. Gottman (2023)

References

Bradbury, T. N., & Bodenmann, G. (2020). Interventions for couples. *Annual Review of Clinical Psychology, 16,* 99–123.

Chapman, G. (1996). *The Five Love Languages: How to Express Heartfelt Commitment to your Mate.* Moody Publishers.

Conradi, H. J., Noordhof, A. & Arntz, A. (2020) Improvement of conflict handling: Hand-holding during and after conflict discussions affects heart rate, mood, and observed communication behavior in romantic partners, *Journal of Sex & Marital Therapy, 46,* 419–434, DOI: 10.1080/0092623X.2020.1748778

Davis, D. E., Yang, X., DeBlaere, C., McElroy, S. E., Van Tongeren, D. R., Hook, J. N., & Worthington, E. L., Jr. (2016). The Injustice Gap. *Psychology of Religion and Spirituality, 8*(3), 175–184. https://doi.org/10.1037/rel0000042

Duong, M. (2023, March 29). Five ways to have more constructive disagreements. *Greater Good Magazine.* Retrieved July 14, 2023, from https://greatergood.berkeley.edu/article/item/five_ways_to_have_more_constructive_disagreements

Fisher, R., Ury, W. L., & Patton. B. (2011). *Getting to Yes: Negotiating Agreement Without Giving In.* Penguin Books.

Gordon, A. M., Impett, E. A., Kogan, A., Oveis, C., & Keltner, D. (2012). To have and to hold: Gratitude promotes relationship maintenance in intimate bonds. *Journal of Personality and Social Psychology, 103*(2), 257–274. https://doi.org/10.1037/a0028723

Gottman, J. M. (1993). A theory of marital dissolution and stability: Families in transition. *Journal of Family Psychology,* 7(1), 57–75.

Gottman, J. M. (2011). *The science of trust: Emotional attunement for couples* (First edition.). W. W. Norton.

Gottman, J. M., & Gottman, J. S. (2015). *Gottman couple therapy.* In A. S. Gurman, J. L. Lebow, & D. S. Snyder (Eds.), *Clinical handbook of couple therapy* (pp. 129–157). Guilford Press.

Gottman, J. M., & Gottman, J. S. (2023). The Gottman method couple therapy. In J. L. Lebow & D. K. Snyder (Eds.), *Clinical handbook of couple therapy, 6th ed.* (pp. 362–386). The Guilford Press.

Gronchi, G., & Giovanelli, F. (2018). Dual process theory of thought and default mode network: A possible neural foundation of fast thinking. *Frontiers in Psychology, 9,* https://doi.org/10.3389/fpsyg.2018.01237

Guerin, P. J., Jr., Fogarty, T. F., Fay, L. F., & Kautto, J. G. (1996). *Working with Relationship Triangles: The One-Two-Three of Psychotherapy.* Guilford Press.

Kahneman, D. (2011). *Thinking, Fast and Slow.* Farrar, Straus, Giroux.

[Praxis CET]. (2023, January 21). *Drop the Rope ACT Exercise by Steven C. Hayes* [Video]. YouTube. www.youtube.com/watch?v=bKx7_Eqimlk

14 Promoting Better Communication

Facilitate What They Already Know

Problem:	Communication interventions are common, but why they work isn't understood.
Solution:	Reflect on three theories of communication in the goals of communication interventions with couples.

In researching this book, Jen and Ev listened to dozens of podcasts, TEDx talks, and conference speakers on couple counseling. Almost all of them had great ideas that helped their couples, and most wanted to help couples communicate. After all, communication is couple's #1 request for help.

In all of those talks, well over 75 percent gave no indication that they had a theory of communication or a theory of change. One speaker began their first session by teaching active listening. Then, throughout the one-hour talk, couples were to be encouraged to paraphrase what their partner had said. What was the theory of change that was implicit and never labeled? We don't know because he never said. We think everyone needs to dig deeper to understand the assumptions behind their communication techniques.

How You Understand Communication Helps You Select Communication Techniques

There are three types of theories of communication. One emphasizes the semantics, the second, syntax; the third, the pragmatics of communication.

Semantics theories of communication

Semantics involve whether the meaning of a communication is clearly communicated and understood. This sees poor transmission or reception

DOI: 10.4324/9781003009382-16

of communication as the problem. The counselor's goal is to help partners clarify communication. This was the focus of the webinar playlist by Dawn-Elise Snipes (Snipes, 2022). Couple counseling was, of course, responsive to whatever the partners brought up, but the theory of counseling was that change in the relationship would occur when couples communicated clearly and responded accurately. With that basis, it was assumed that partners could work out all relational differences.

Couple therapists who hold a semantics view of communication use methods that help partners understand the meaning of the other person and clearly express their own meaning. Their theory of change is that if people know each other's meanings, they will communicate well. So, therapy helps partners clarify their own meanings and understand their partner's meanings. These methods include techniques that promote active listening, teach and communicate empathy, and help couples decode nonverbal communication that qualifies their verbalizations and can contaminate or enhance understanding.

Syntax theories of communication

Syntax involves the way people punctuate their interactions. It's not what partners say or don't say that causes communication snafus. It's how they do or don't say it. Do they insert a question mark regarding each other's commitment and good intentions? Do they yell, placing exclamation marks on topics that disturb them? Do they speak in run-on sentences, with one person dominating and seeming to talk non-stop? Or do they rarely speak, yielding pages of blank copy, withdrawing, and disengaging?

Couple therapists who believe that the essence of communication is syntactic patterns of communication seek to identify and change systemic patterns of communication—preferably to some pattern that is more functional. They see those stable patterns of poor syntax as the cause of problems. They use many methods to break up negative communication patterns (i.e., interrupt the usual syntax). They tend to be less concerned with building good patterns of communication. The implicit message is that poor patterns are problematic. There are many functional ways of communicating, so let's break up the old way and then see if the new way is more functional.

The idea is similar to Jay Haley's demonstration (based on Haley, 1963, and elaborated in Haley, 1976) in which he would tip a chair over on its side to represent a stable, nonfunctional system. He would lift the chair until it was balanced on one or two legs, saying that the couple must pass through an unstable state (never meant to be the end-point) in order to get to a stable, functional system. Thus, he would try to disrupt old interaction patterns, not concerned about the unstable new situation. He then moved the partners to some stable but functional structure.

Pragmatics theories of communication

Pragmatics involves the subtext of communications. What effects do the communications have (Watzawick et al., 2011/1967)? Often, the effects have to do with what a partner believes empowers him or her. For example, one couple might have a wife who seems to talk incessantly and a husband who only talks about significant matters. The wife might believe that by controlling the flow and content of almost every conversation, she has the power in the relationship. When she feels anxious, she talks even more and may talk over her partner. The husband might believe that his wife prattles on about nothing, but he has the power because he can have a say about the "important" issues in the relationship. When he feels anxious, he tends to shut down or, alternatively, he defines this issue as "important," and he demands that his wife listen and obey because this is his area of expertise.

Couple therapists who emphasize pragmatics look for the effects that communication patterns have. These effects might be simple—like a man who comes home from work anticipating conflict with his wife might move directly to his room, to the television set, to internet pornography, or to the refrigerator for the first of many cocktails. Behavior therapists who do functional analyses are taking a pragmatics approach. They try to help partners develop other patterns of behavior that have desired, not pernicious, effects on the relationship. Power struggles (see Haley, 1976), as we saw in the previous chapter, are thought to be not disagreement over content but over who has the authority to decide. That is a pragmatic interpretation of a power struggle.

Communication can be analyzed from any of those vantage points

Note that any pattern of behavior can be interpreted as a problem of semantics, syntax, or pragmatics. So, a therapist holding a semantics view of a power struggle sees the ways that partners fail to understand each other. They interrupt the power struggle to have partners stop, say what they want clearly, reflect back on what the partner said, and work on a common understanding.

A therapist holding a syntax view of the same power struggle might not care how they did it, but they would try to break up the patterns—the usual ways of acting. The therapist believes that, if they did so, the power struggle would be averted. Therapists might observe that the wife tries to overpower the husband with many words, and the husband gets angry because he doesn't feel heard. So, the therapists might recommend that the wife talk less and the husband lower his demands to be listened to. The syntax-oriented couple therapist is content to break up the old pattern—however, it happens. Then, after the pattern is disrupted, the therapist can suggest a new pattern that is more functional.

Instigating More Positive Communications That Convey Valuing for the Partner

We believe that affectively positive communications are to be encouraged and affectively negative ones to be discouraged. From a semantics viewpoint, positive communications are easier to understand. Communications loaded with negative affect divert attention from understanding and lead to miscommunications. But affectively positive communications also tend to be more often functional in keeping the interactions aimed at accomplishing the tasks of the relationship—i.e., getting the work done in the relationship. But they are also more functional in being less likely to divert conversations into arguing, put-downs, emotional explosions, and negative reciprocity. So, from a syntactical viewpoint, we want to prolong positive patterns of communication and interrupt and change negative dysfunctional patterns. From the pragmatics viewpoint, we believe that the effects of affectively positive communication include conveying that partners value or love each other, which strengthens the emotional bond.

Which is the right way to help people communicate? That is not the important question. If we have learned one thing about couple therapy, it is that it is not what you do that matters as much as what you do about what you do. Any of these approaches might change the pattern of a couple.

But changing patterns of communication isn't the outcome we are searching for. It's a means to the important end of promoting more maturity, stability, and satisfaction by creating, growing, and maintaining a healthy emotional bond. From our perspective, it doesn't matter whether you focus on semantics, syntax, or pragmatics. As long as the work is characterized by valuing love and faith, which leads to hope, that then creates strong bonds and happy outcomes. So, any (tried and true) techniques will help. You can use your favorite or one that uses therapy ju-jitsu and metaphors to support the change. What we do encourage therapists to do is to ponder what your own theory of communication is and how well it fits with the couple in front of you.

Regardless of one's preferred theory of communication, we believe that we should provide opportunities to guide partners into communicating more positively more of the time. Thus, we provide interventions promoting affectively positive communications.

Interventions Promoting Affectively Positive Communications

Initially, couple therapists observed research that showed that couples who had high ratios of positive to negative interactions were more satisfied and less likely to divorce than those with lower ratios. Thus, therapists sought to help couples move their ratios higher by increasing positive interactions and decreasing negative interactions (see Intervention 14-1). This intervention is effective, but not at producing couples that are automatically satisfied and at low risk of divorce. Rather, this intervention does help strengthen the emotional bond.

Intervention 14-1 Love Bank

The therapist describes the couple's relationship as Love Bank. Each positive loving and valuing act is like a deposit of one love-dollar. Each negative act is like a withdrawal of five love-dollars. (This is because negative acts are much more powerful than positive ones; Baumeister, 1998.) Try to keep a positive balance in both partners' love banks.

We often use this love-bank intervention early in counseling when conflict is still high to redirect couples toward what they can do to repair the emotional bond instead of one-upping the partner or merely defending themselves (see Intervention 14-2). Spend time in session helping the couple plan weekly dates, check-ins, and random acts of kindness, then working through reluctance and resistance to this kind of change. And encourage partners to keep their own bank balance, not their partner's.

Couples have modified the Love Bank for their own preferences. Intervention 14-2 provides spin-off love-bank interventions.

Intervention 14-2 Love Bank Spin-Offs

We have used several modifications of the Love Bank.

- Track positives and give yourselves a gold star or $5 for each, and then use the reward to party on and do something fun for a date together.
- Creating a Love-Bank "jar" with positive deposit ideas written on the list.
- Having the couple keep a log or journal of love-bank deposits (but not withdrawals) during the week to focus them on positive interactions.

- Use websites or smartphone apps for ideas, and keep lists and reminders in an electronic calendar to make specific love-bank deposits.
- Social media like Pinterest, websites, and apps are full of ideas to improve one's relationship that fits the love-bank genre. Get inspired by other couples' ideas.

Interventions Promoting Changes in the Way Partners Typically Communicate

These interventions are formalized ways of helping partners communicate the way they would like to communicate. Four will be taken as examples.

Listen and repeat

The first is to listen and repeat what is said (described in the LOVE Intervention 13-1). This typically appeals to clinicians who favor a semantics approach because the rationale that is given is usually to help partners better understand their meanings. But, as we know, the formality of the intervention also breaks up the patterns (i.e., syntax) and assumes an underlying meaning of valuing the partner (i.e., pragmatics). This is our "go-to" intervention for couples who can do little else for communication other than listen and repeat. The hope is that their hurting selves will experience valuing and work in the intervention to repair their bond.

Active listening

Dysregulated couples tend to discount their partner and passively (or not at all) respond to each other. The speaker-listener technique (see Intervention 14-3) involves some work for couples but is quite simple. It can increase their faith in therapy, lead to hope, and increase their bond.

Intervention 14-3 Making Affirming Active Responses Using the Speaker–Listener Technique

One partner discusses a life triumph or struggle other than the relationship. The listener is coached to respond in ways that are both affirming and active. The opposite of positive active responding is disengaged and discounting. We find that it fits especially well as part of the weekly homework for couples who would like to connect more deeply.

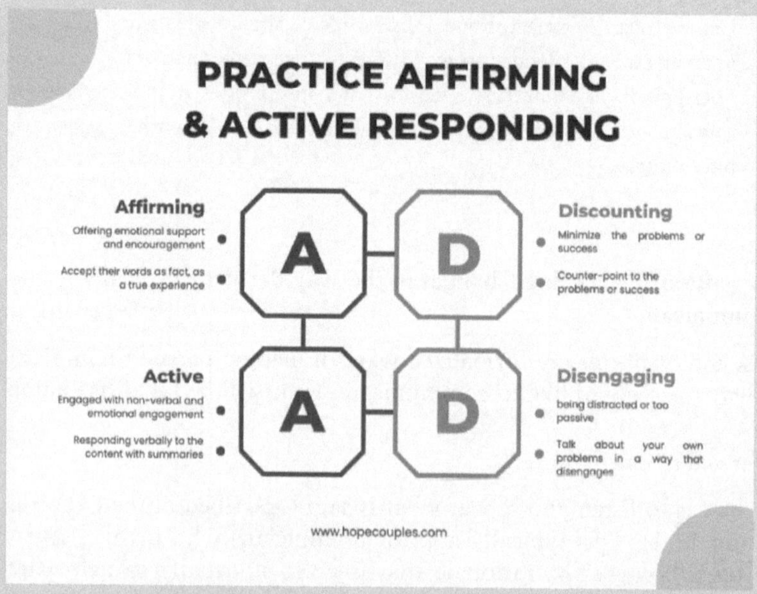

Figure 14-1 Practice Affirming and Active Responding Instead of Discounting and Disengaging

One couple had a breakthrough using this intervention when the therapist said that affirming doesn't mean happy-clappy. Instead, affirming has two definitions: to state something is a fact and to offer support to someone. One wife was discussing her struggles with an anxiety disorder while pregnant and unable to take her usual medications. Her wife was uncomfortable with the anxiety disorder and often afraid it would be directed at her. She had tried to cope with both their discomfort by attempting to cheer her partner up and fix the unsolvable problem, which had only made them both feel worse. After this communication session, she moved towards her wife with a listening ear, *affirmed* her experience, and *actively* joined her in her sadness.

Leveling and editing

In the couple clinic at Regent University, we have used leveling and editing heavily (see Intervention 14-4). *Leveling* is saying what one needs to say in a way that can be received without self-censorship. Leveling is often very important for partners who tend to withdraw or hide their emotions. *Editing* is being able to control oneself emotionally when tempted to a harmful outburst. A partner is often so angry, so sad, or so overwhelmed that they are emotionally drowning and dragging their partner along with them. Many approaches coach in emotion regulation, such as self-soothing in Gottman therapy, too-much-emotion problems in emotionally focused therapy, emotion-regulation skills in dialectical behavior therapy, and defocusing in acceptance and commitment therapy. You'll notice that this is heavy in a syntactical approach to communication.

Intervention 14-4 Leveling and Editing

This intervention is usually triggered when a partner, or both, is either keeping secrets or losing emotional control and blasting the partner. Describe both leveling and editing and give an example of each. Analyze the communication that triggered the use of the intervention using the relevant concept.

For leveling, have partners practice a soft start-up (Intervention 13-11). For editing, coach partners to pause before responding, lower emotion through long out-breaths, then focus attention on internal experiences.

Identify triggers (aka "love busters")

The love-busters intervention (see Intervention 14-5) encourages couples to identify negative triggers that they say or do in their relationship (see Harley, 2016). Partners think through hurtful things they have used more than once. These are referred to as "love busters." Merely identifying triggers can be important. The idea is to break up those love-busting patterns. So, this typically appeals to couple therapists who value syntactical interventions.

Because this technique is based on the idea that awareness will change behavior, it works best for couples who are either early in their relationship or not entrenched in high-octane negative reciprocity. It may seem that doing "Love Busters" with high conflict would match their needs, but our experience has shown that partners who have trouble controlling emotional conflict have practiced patterns that make awareness-based interventions ineffective. Also, such couples often use what they learn through this exercise as ammunition for their next battle.

Intervention 14-5 Love Busters

- The therapist names patterns that inflict hurt, "love busters."
- Give examples. Common ones are, "You always ignore me," or "You're selfish, just like your father!", "I'm leaving you" or simply refusing to talk/stone-walling.

- Ask partners to identify anything they know they have said to the partner that had a particularly hurtful effect. (We start with partners reflecting on their own behavior rather than beginning with accusations.)
- Ask the partner whether there are other things that were especially hurtful that should be avoided.

If the love-busters intervention succeeds, the couples identifying love-busting as a problem will reduce their attacks and put-downs.

Use speaker-listener structures

We have asked couples in the Hope couples lab since 2012 which interventions they found most helpful to them. Of all the ones listed, the TANGO (see Intervention 14-6) is consistently #1. It might be something about the memorability of the intervention, which involves standing and a simple but practical experience of communication that pulls together the basic principles of relating well as a couple. It is one of our central speaker–listener communication interventions. As one of the couples commented, "While it's just a tool, it's a really useful one!"

Intervention 14-6 TANGO and TANGO-E

TANGO

Stand. The couple is asked to stand up. This makes the intervention more memorable and engages their whole body in remembering how to change communication patterns. Couples who sit tend to fall into old patterns of speaker–speaker, while those standing tend to be able to engage the speaker–listener goals. For telehealth modality, we have tried the sitting modality so we could hear and see the couple more clearly. However, we still believe that standing is essential, and while it may require some work on the part of the couple to stand up in front of the camera, it is well worth it. If standing is not possible, ask them to find a small object that the listener will hold as a reminder not to talk back until the listener's turn.

The order. The speaker in the TANGO is responsible for the TAN.

T: *Tell* what happened, directly and briefly. A few minutes, not more.

A: Explain how it *Affected* you. (Sometimes an emotion-words chart is helpful.)

N: *Nurturing* statement. Say something you love about your partner.

The listener is responsible for the GO.

G: *Get* it? The listener summarizes what they heard and asks, "Did I get it?"

O: *Observe* the effects of the conversation. (This is the O in the LOVE acronym, Intervention 13–1.) The listener is also responsible for observing how the conversation is going and whether they are communicating well as a couple.[1]

Resistances. It's common for listeners to want to jump to the speaker role, arguing back before the speaker has finished talking. When that happens, it's an opportunity to reflect on their natural motivations to "get you to understand *me*" rather than to focus on what the other is saying. This is a courageous act of faith that they can get their turn to express themselves. Also, they explicitly say something loving about the partner (the N, Nurturing statement). Finally, the act of listening is a statement that they value the partner.

When finished with the exercise, the therapist shares the hidden "rules" of the intervention, which are the important principles of communication to apply even if they do not use TANGO at home. Those principles are:

1. Take turns being the leader who is speaking. Only one speaker at a time.
2. Be brief when you are the speaker.
3. Don't try to solve problems. Slow down. Work to understand the other person's perspective, feelings, and hopes.
4. If either of you feel emotionally flooded, take a break and cool down.
5. Affection, valuing statements, and a tender touch are needed. They communicate more than words.

TANGO-E

The TANGO intervention is supplemented by adding the E ("Evaluating Underlying Interests") portion of the LOVE intervention (Intervention 13–1). For partners who need to solve a solvable problem, TANGO carries them through listening. Then they take another turn as speaker and then listener in which they share their best understanding of their underlying interests. This sets them up to make good decisions together as a couple. TANGO-E also shortens the time spent on communication plus conflict resolution.

Avoid high-stress problem solving

Have you ever noticed how many arguments seem to happen when one or both partners is exhausted or stressed to the max? There is a good reason. Stress requires self-control, and (I know that this shocks you) self-control exhausts our innate coping resources. Roy Baumeister and his colleagues showed that doing a self-control task reduced performance on a subsequent self-control task. Baumeister and others (Baumeister et al., 2007; Hagger et al., 2016) have supported this in a multitude of studies. But Baumeister also showed that something sugary could replace some of the stress-exhausted glucose in our brain (Gailliot & Baumeister, 2007). Intervention 14-7 gives some ways to prevent being sidetracked by exhaustion.

Intervention 14-7 A Coke and a Smile

Ask couples to:

- Notice common situations and times when they are likely too tired or stressed for deep and emotion-filled conversations. For example, after 10pm, after an exhausting day at work, or even after a long weekend, cheering for their son's soccer tournament, are unlikely times to successfully resolve a conflict.
- Partners negotiate a plan for how they will ask each other to delay difficult conversations for a better time. This is similar to the time-out principle and an important self-control task in and of itself.
- This intervention can also uncover chronic exhaustion, trauma reactivity, or deeper patterns of avoidance in the couple. These more stable negative communication patterns may need more intensive attention in treatment to see progress.
- Even some therapy activities like Processing Conflict (see Intervention 13–10) or TANGO (see Intervention 14–6) are ill-advised when they are tired.
- They might also notice that if they attend a couple of therapy sessions when they are tired and stressed, they have fewer resources to process their relationship during sessions. Planning their schedule to be able to give their "best selves" to their therapy helps the process go more effectively and quickly (and therefore less costly, too!)

Conclusion

Let's put a closing punctuation on communication. Most people who attend couple therapy say they want to improve their communication. Sometimes, that's a catch-all word to mean that they are in pain, stressed out, and feel ineffective in reaching their goal of a peaceful, loving, and stable relationship. Communication techniques meet the couple where they are, prioritizing their needs and requests. Anytime we can directly address their desire for a better communication pattern and walk away at the end of the session where they say, "Ya know, that went better than usual for our communication. I think I understand you better and feel understood," then we have sparked hope. We only need a demonstration of good communication to create a small spark to bond a couple together.

It is easy to wrongly believe that communication techniques have some kind of power for change or that communication is itself the problem. They do not and it is not. Instead, they kick off a cycle that works to help restore emotional bonds. A good bond is the seedbed for the outcomes we are all searching for in close relationships: stability, maturity, and satisfaction. Good conflict resolution and communication that uses a strategy of faith, work, and love will increase hope that their pain will be replaced with the longed-for relationship of their dreams. Once you have them hoping, they will work harder and with more courage for the relationship dreams to come true.

Note

1 A worksheet, blog post, and video demonstrations of TANGO can be found at hopecouples.com

References

Baumeister R. F. (1998). The self. In D. T. Gilbert, S. T. Fiske, & G. Lindzey, *Handbook of Social Psychology (4th ed.),* (pp. 680–740). McGraw-Hill.

Baumeister, R. F., Vohs, K. D., & Tice, D. M. (2007). The strength model of self-control. *Current Directions in Psychological Science, 16*, 351–355.

Gailliot, M. T., & Baumeister, R. F. (2007). The physiology of willpower: Linking blood glucose to self-control. *Personality and Social Psychology Review, 11*(4), 303–327. https://doi.org/10.1177/1088868307303030

Hagger, M. S., Chatzisarantis, N. L. D., Alberts, H., Anggono, C. O., Batailler, C., . . . & Zwienenberg, M. (2016). A multilab pre-registered replication of the ego depletion effect. *Perspectives on Psychological Science, 11*(4), 546–573.

Haley, J. (1963). *Strategies of Psychotherapy*. Grune & Stratton.

Haley, J. (1976). *Problem-Solving Therapy*. San Francisco, CA: Jossey-Bass.

Harley, W. F. (2016). *Love Busters*. Revell.

Snipes, D. E. (2022, October 27). *Doc Snipes' practical tools for health and happiness*. Doc Snipes YouTube Channel. Retrieved July 17, 2023, from https://www.youtube.com/playlist?list=PLcB3trehXswjMw_Wpxn_8BGAD-vN9DVgw

Watzlawick, P., Bavelas, J. B., & Jackson, D. D. (2011/1967). *The Pragmatics of Human Communication: A Study of Interactional Patterns, Pathologies, and Paradoxes*. W. W. Norton (originally published 1967).

Part 3

Bonding

15 Revealing the Secret to a Happy Romantic Relationship

Help Build a More Intimate Emotional Bond

Problem:	Couples long for a warm supportive emotional bond, yet they struggle to create one.
Solution:	Employ gentle, but effective interventions that create a safe supportive bond.

The Pushkin podcast "Deep Cover" tells the fascinating story of Esther Reed (Halpern, 2023), a chameleon who lived a double life full of loneliness, crime, and tragedy. At 21, she suddenly disappeared from her small town and dysfunctional family. Locals believed she had been kidnapped or murdered. But she was alive.

She cut ties with everyone she knew and created a new identity. Walking away from a tragic childhood is familiar enough, but Esther took the unusual path of stealing identities to earn college credit. She attended Harvard and Columbia University and earned 1400 on the SAT despite being a high school dropout. She dated a Naval Academy cadet for some time and then disappeared suddenly when her identity was discovered, spending years alone on the run. Her history caught the attention of authorities, who put her on the FBI most-wanted list, thinking she might be involved in espionage.

Aware of the dragnet, Esther hid for years. She had no friends. She hid from authorities and survived on her huckster abilities. In the Deep Cover interview, Esther describes a romantic relationship with the Naval cadet as a brief respite of relief in a life of isolation, identity theft, and scamming. She describes relating to his kind and welcoming family as a bizarre experience. How can a normal dating relationship be bizarre to a woman in her 20s?

Much has been written about attachment theory as the basis for understanding human relationships (Arriaga et al., 2018). We agree that attachment bond is foundational. The sad story of the lonely Esther Reed is a

DOI: 10.4324/9781003009382-18

cautionary tale. Finding a healthy primary attachment relationship is a necessary foundation for a good life. Losing a vital bond starts many tragic narratives. Babies need good parents, teens need good friends, and adults need a healthy bond with a partner. Without these, life can be hard.

In this chapter, we discuss five types of couple bonds—sexual, emotional, social, intellectual, and recreational—that build most healthily from secure attachment. We describe a triangular interdependence model of satisfaction and commitment (Sternberg, 1986). The interventions based on that model seek to help couples build more intimacy, share passion, and reinforce commitments in ways that are congruent with their individual and partnership attachment needs.

Usable Theories

Sternberg's triangular theory of love

Sternberg (1986) crafted a triangular theory of love. Love has three parts: passion, intimacy, and commitment. If we think of each being either high or low, a taxonomy of eight types of love would emerge (see Figure 15-1).

1 Mature love is high in all three. (Sternberg labeled it consummate love.) Mature love would be an excellent outcome of couple therapy and is the unstated goal of most couples.
2 Infatuation is high in passion and low in intimacy and commitment. This is usually the first type of love in a romantic relationship. Infatuation fuels early adult attachment.
3 When intimacy is high but passion and commitment are low, partners tend to like each other and may be "best friends."
4 Empty love relationships retain commitment but have low levels of passion and intimacy. Such love leads partners to feel like roommates. They often have low sexual contact and live separate disconnected lives.
5 Romantic love is high in intimacy and passion, but commitment is low. This phase occurs for most relationships as they continue to date or even slide into living together.
6 Fatuous (e.g., foolish) love is high in passion and commitment but low in intimacy. Such couples jump directly from passionate attraction to a silly, too-early commitment in which intimacy has not yet begun to grow. They might get tattoos of each other's names, move in together, or marry after only knowing each other briefly.
7 Companionate love find that passion fires lose intensity. The relationship is one of intimacy and commitment devoid of passion. Sternberg

(1986) suggests that most healthy couples spend many years emphasizing friendship and commitment, but they often have lost passion.

8 Non-love would be low in all three. The non-love couple is quite hopeless if they seek couple therapy.

Classifying relationships according to this taxonomy might help partners and therapists decide what aspects they want to work on in couple therapy. The most frequent couples seeking couple therapy are those with non-love (i.e., our relationship is lifeless), companionate love (i.e., our passion is gone), or even liking (we still have a sense of intimacy, but it is more like friendship in which our passion and commitment are waning or absent).

We have found it helpful, especially during the initial assessment, to have partners plot the relative height of each aspect of their love over different phases of their relationship (see Intervention 15-1). This theory is readily understood, and couples can often identify other aspects of their relationship as a simple type of processing the relationship.

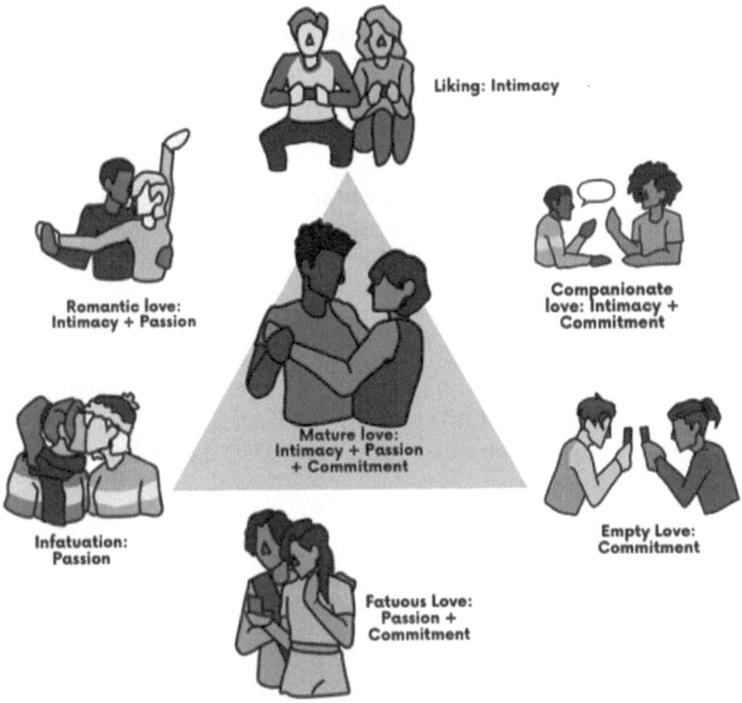

Figure 15-1 Sternberg's Eight Types of Love Derived from Being High or Low in Passion, Intimacy, and Commitment

Intervention 15-1 Plot the Couple's Sternberg Love-Triangle History

Couples make a time-line (horizontal axis) beginning at the time of their meeting. They create three lines—one for each type of love (passion, intimacy, and commitment). They can note significant relationship events to show how the level of each component of love (on the vertical axis) might have changed with events. In session, this can generate good discussions.

Interdependence theory of satisfaction and commitment

Theories of love are a helpful, developmentally informed way to get a handle on a relationship. It doesn't explain the dynamic, ever-changing interplay that describes how a couple relates. For help understanding the emotional bond, we turn to interdependence theory. Interdependence theory has extensive research support with over 1000 studies to provide a versatile and dynamic framework to understand how two people relate (Johnson & Johnson, 2006; Kelley & Thibaut, 1978). This theory emphasizes positive or negative actions and processes that explain patterns of cooperation or opposition, which leads to achieving or being thwarted from goals.

Interdependence theory and its outgrowth, the investment model of commitment (Rusbult, 1980), proposes that individuals are more committed to and dependent upon the relationship to the extent that:

1 The relationship is satisfying.
2 There are high perceived rewards relative to costs.
3 Partners have made investments (i.e., time, tangible resources, energy, responsibilities, shared memories, or children) in the relationship.
4 Alternatives to the relationship (i.e., aloneness, different partner, career) are relatively poor.

A meta-analysis of 52 studies revealed that these factors predict commitment to romantic partners, friends, family, and work (Le & Agnew, 2003). Commitment, in turn, predicts many pro-relationship behaviors, including accommodation (turning the other cheek), sacrifice (forgoing one's self-interest for the partner's benefit), and forgiveness (Finkel et al., 2002).

According to the theory, a person may be dissatisfied with the relationship, yet committed to it if investments are high and alternatives unsatisfactory (Rusbult, 1980). So, unsatisfying or abusive relationships may persist over time, with or without forgiveness, because commitment or dependence is high.

Dependence on the partner gives the partner *power*, which is the ability to influence relationship outcomes. Typically, commitment and dependence are highly correlated in partners. This interdependence theory analysis of power as equal to the partner's dependence yields a counter-intuitive conclusion. Power is *not* a zero-sum game in relationships. Levels of dependence of each party typically are positively rather than negatively correlated. Thus, when people are highly committed to the relationship and each other, they also exert power over each other. A committed partner has the power to ask for big things, like moving cross-country for a job or having a baby sooner than initially planned. Power is characterized by three types of control: actor control, partner control, and joint control.

1. *Actor control* is one partner's ability to control their outcomes. If one's partner (call her Jean) influences her own outcomes, that is actor control. Jean decides to purchase some new clothes with her funds, which would be actor control.
2. When Jean's behaviors influence the other's (call her LaShawn) outcomes, then LaShawn is experiencing *partner control*. For example, if Jean decides where the couple will vacation regardless of what LaShawn wants, then LaShawn is experiencing partner control.
3. *Joint control* means that the choices of both partners determine the outcomes of both partners. For example, Jean prefers eating Chinese food. LaShawn likes eating Italian food. Yet both partners would be more dissatisfied eating alone than eating what the partner prefers. They have joint control over each other's choices, and they can make choices so that both are satisfied.

If Jean has power over LaShawn, then Jean can make more selfish behavioral choices that reduce LaShawn's relationship satisfaction. But Jean does not have unlimited power. She cannot make choices that would reduce LaShawn's satisfaction below the point in which LaShawn can get better outcomes from an *alternative* to their relationship. In that case, LaShawn would, if things could not be changed, end the relationship if possible. At a minimum, she would withdraw and reduce the interdependence, opting for more independence.

If LaShawn believes she has few options for alternative relationships, she will be more likely to forgive or reconcile if Jean hurts or offends her. On the other hand, Jean will be less likely to apologize, make amends, seek forgiveness, or move toward reconciliation if she believes LaShawn is stuck in the relationship with few alternatives. Therapists need a good conceptualization to assist the couple in how to use their power for the good of their relationship (see Intervention 15-2).

Intervention 15-2 Conceptualization of Three Types of Power

Knowing these types of power from interdependence theory, you can use your observations of types of power, of satisfaction, commitment, and willingness to sacrifice as guideposts to select interventions that will help the couple move courageously toward their relationship goals. You can encourage them to relinquish exercising power by domination that builds dependence. You can encourage them to share power, build satisfaction (rewards vs costs, low satisfaction with alternatives), increase commitment (increased satisfaction and investments, lower satisfaction with alternatives).

Interventions to Assess and Build Intimacy

Assess different types of intimacy

Let's face it. There might be no limit to the types of intimacy people experience, and what makes one person feel intimate might make another feel creepy. But we need to narrow the field to some kinds of intimacy that seem common, are easy to assess, and provide fruitful targets for intervention. Mark Schaefer and David Olson (1981) created the Pair Inventory, which identified and evaluated the ideal and experienced amount of five types of intimacy experienced. Intimacy was seen as closeness, the bond that glues a relationship together, and includes feelings of safety, security, attachment, and love. Each type of intimacy should be assessed individually rather than aggregated. Because Schaefer and Olson's instrument is unavailable, we adapted a simple visual analog to assess the five types of intimacy—marking on five intimacy thermometers what the current and ideal amount of each type is (see Intervention 15-3).

1 *Emotional intimacy* is the feeling that one is emotionally close to the partner and able to share essential emotions. It includes trust.
2 *Sexual intimacy* is the closeness one feels in relating sexually to the partner. It is not just having sex, though that is important. It includes vulnerability and trust in opening oneself sexually to the partner.
3 *Social intimacy* is closeness in sharing types and amounts of social activities.
4 *Intellectual intimacy* is the closeness in sharing talk about ideas and concepts.

5 *Recreational intimacy* is closeness regarding how partners spend their time recreationally in sports, games, and pastimes?

Bonus: *Spiritual intimacy* is not explicitly included in Schaeffer and Olson's taxonomy. However, for highly religious or spiritual couples, their value on the spiritual life and perhaps religious activities may bond them. This may include organized religious activities, individual or couple-oriented spiritual disciplines, or spirituality (e.g., yoga, time in nature, etc.), which makes it worth assessing separately for some.

Intervention 15-3 Assess and Process the Intimacy Thermometers

We assess five types of intimacy using intimacy thermometers (rated from 0 to 100). We prefer to ask partners to mark their ideal and current experienced intimacy for each of the five (or six, if spiritual intimacy seems as if it will be important to the couple). While there is no psychometric support for the reliability or validity of these thermometers, there is excellent clinical utility and the face validity is high—couples treat the measures as accurate.

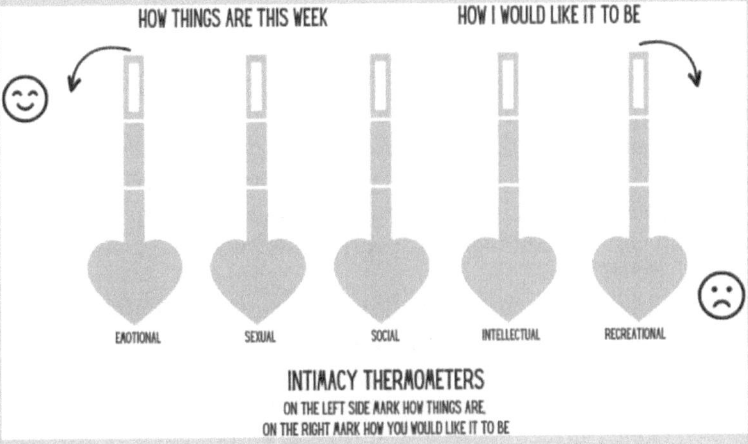

Figure 15-2 Intimacy Thermometers (Ripley & Worthington, 2014)

Graph emotional closeness throughout the history of the relationship

If you have asked couples to complete the intimacy thermometers (Intervention 15-3; see Figure 15-2) at the beginning of each session, you can graph any particular type of intimacy that is relevant for treatment (see Intervention 15-4). Because each thermometer is rated on the same response metric, from 0 to 100, you could display all types of intimacy over time by using the same graph. This same method can be used to retrospectively rate intimacy at different important times in the history of the relationship.

Intervention 15-4 Graphing Closeness Throughout the Relationship

When couples arrive at the beginning of each session, provide a hard copy for each of the types of intimacy using intimacy thermometers (see Figure 15-2). When it suits your treatment purpose, you can create a session-by-session graph of the ratings of the type of intimacy under consideration. This works well to introduce and track interventions on sexual intimacy and bonding in particular.

Communicate about love languages to build intimacy through better communication

Pastor Gary Chapman (1992) suggested that there are five primary "love languages" that people prefer. Although this began as a Christian book, it has transcended cultural barriers and is familiar to most people regardless of religion or secular status (Chapman, 2023). There are over 20M in print, translated into 49 languages. This is now a cottage industry with resources for love languages for children, military personnel, singles, workplace colleagues, and for apologizing. Some tests assess one's love languages and partner's love languages.

According to Chapman, the five love languages are physical touch and closeness, acts of service, gift-giving, quality time, and words of affirmation. The claim is that communicating in the partner's primary love language will yield greater relationship success. Gery Karantzas (2023) recently observed in *Greater Good Magazine* that the concept is supported by research. Four studies tested a central claim that partners matched on love language are more satisfied. Three early studies were weakly supportive but the most recent are more firmly supportive. Two studies supported the claim that knowing a partner's love language resulted in higher partner satisfaction. Factor analytic studies suggest Chapman's five love languages exist, but there might be others. Many claims made in the popular press are never scientifically investigated. So, it is encouraging that at least some scientific attention has been given and that the few studies available are cautiously supportive. At a minimum, love languages provide a conversation starter and focus for couples (see Intervention 15-5).

Intervention 15-5 Five Love Languages to Increase Emotional Bonds

The five love languages can help couples increase their bond.

- Introduce the concept. If partners have not heard of the love languages, give them a brief summary and mention that some research supports their use in couples. If they are interested refer them to the *Greater Good Magazine* article by Karantzas (2023).
- Use homework to Google the love languages, find a test to assess each of theirs, and discuss their findings after each takes the test.
- Talk in session about what they found.
- Ask partners to identify what they intend to do to communicate more in the partner's primary love language.

Sculpting intimacy

Because we seek to make change "sensible" with each intervention, it is not surprising that we use sculpting within interventions to promote intimacy, conflict resolution, communication, and forgiveness and reconciliation. In sculpting, you ask a partner to use their own body and their partner's body to represent symbolically what is being experienced (see Intervention 15-6). There is a demonstration of a couple in counseling with Ev using sculpting with a forgiveness issue on the Hope website.[1] The uses of sculpting to reflect different adaptive and maladaptive couple experiences on intimacy are almost unlimited.

The mechanics of creating this intervention are as flexible as the number of sculptures that can be made. Here are a few ideas for the use of sculptures.

- **Individual assessment.** Partners take turns to show intimacy or strong emotion.
- **Diagnosis of ability to compromise.** Couples seek to create a compromise sculpture. That shows how they work together and compromise, or don't. So, it can often be used in the section on conflict resolution.

- **Agreeing on hopes and dreams.** Couples can create an ideal sculpture to represent ideal intimacy, communication, conflict resolution, and forgiveness, either together or as individuals.
- **A stimulus for a discussion about how to change intimacy.** The couple can create a sculpture to model something like "the way you see the relationship today." (Sometimes, partners might ask the therapist to use one of their phones to take a picture.) Once the sculpture is complete, the therapist can seat the partners and ask questions for discussion. For example, "What would help to improve this sculpture to something happier, less tense, more respectful of each other, etc.?" Or "What should we do today to change this sculpture to be more what you would like it to be?"
- **Demonstrating that they are changing.** Sculpting a similar stimulus (i.e., "Sculpt the way you see the intimacy between you today") across sessions can show whether partners are changing their perceptions of intimacy (see Intervention 15-6). Some couples might take a picture of their sculpture each week as a concrete encouragement that their relationship is changing. Such pictures have been used in final-session graduation memorials.

Intervention 15-6 A Sculpting Intervention to Deepen Intimacy Over Time

Ask the couple to use the space in the room. Ask each partner in turn to create a sculpture with their bodies to show the effects of communication on the partners' sense of intimacy. For example, tell the couple, "Create a sculpture of the two of you seeking to act intimately after poor communication; after good communication, what were the differences you tried to get across with your sculptures?"

It's often surprising what couples will do with this intervention. One couple was fighting in session. When asked to create a demonstration with their bodies to sculpt what was happening between them, one partner curled up in a ball on the floor, and the other partner sat in a chair with their head hanging low in their hands. This shocked the therapist because the couple had been hostile and argumentative for half the session. The sculpting allowed the couple to reveal their more vulnerable underlying feelings that were unstated in their "tornado-like" arguing. This "curled up and exhausted" metaphor became a tool to help the couple soften for weeks after that intervention. They could support the "curled up and exhausted" part of each other.

Refocus on Dreams, Hopes, and Solutions Rather than Problems

Solution-focused therapy has an excellent idea worth adopting. Focus on solutions instead of problems.

Solutions help couples solve things while problem-rumination does not. Our approach is not completely oriented toward solutions (as solution-focused therapy seems to be) and away from problems. However, research on change processes and our observations have found that most couples who come to therapy seem intent on recounting their problems to engage the therapist on their side. If you know systems language, this is triangulation. At a minimum, both partners want to tell their slant on the relationship *problems*. They mistakenly believe that telling the problem in front of an objective therapist will irrationally induce their partner to say, "Oh wow. You are right; I have been just awful. You explained all my faults, problems, and failures so well that I will change forever." While it's *possible* some partner somewhere in the world has responded to relationship problems this way, we think we'd be better advised to invest in lottery tickets than in such a wager. Most people change when they focus on winsome visions of how things could be better. The draw of the better hoped-for future fuels long-term change more effectively than problem rehearsal or rumination.

Mapping where the couple wants to go—their dreams, hopes, and specific goals—is not easy (see Intervention 15-7). Most couples have lost hope and have not thought about their dreams and hopes for their relationship for a long time. The therapist, with sensitivity to timing that balances hearing the problems with looking forward, can help the partners to rekindle their hopes and dreams and then devise solutions to get there.

Intervention 15-7 Make Dreams and Hopes Solid

Discussing and negotiating what a perfect relationship might be like can help couples develop a shared meaning for their relationship. Whereas solution-focused therapy tends to focus mostly on the solutions, we move this to a more balanced approach. Partners can not only identify ideal goals but therapists can challenge couples to identify threats and brainstorm how to deal with them. Similarly, the Gottmans have couples discuss their dreams, but the therapist guides the focus on which dreams might be threatened by the partners' distress (Gottman & Gottman, 2023). There are many other variations on how therapists get couples to explore their dreams.

- The therapist asks the couple to create a story of their future as a "perfect" couple with an eye toward their ideal end.

- Often, this can be framed as describing a perfect day in the couple's life.
- One approach can be asking the couple to think about their childhood. What did they think a romantic relationship would be like at that time? Did they hope to find something in their romantic relationship as an adult?
- The partners can recall the origin of their relationship. They describe what attracted them to their partner. They recall (under prompting) the moment when they first believed that their partner loved them and they loved their partner. What fulfillment did they anticipate from that feeling of mutual love?

Partners are asked to determine which of their initial dreams they would still like to pursue and to (informally) prioritize the most important ones.

After partners identify some hopes and dreams worth working for, the therapist might ask each partner if there are any concrete ways that they might do something this week to contribute to meeting the partners' needs.

The therapist looks for themes, such as being loved, finding safety or security, being with someone and not alone, belonging, being understood, getting attention and care, and finding that trust was forming. The therapist helps partners see what types of relational needs they hope will be met. You don't want to be perceived as a cheerleader or motivational speaker. Helping couples see the dreams they want to work toward is a recipe for building hope.

Conclusion

Intimacy interventions have multiple purposes. They are not just intended to make couples feel lovey-dovey. They can be used to assess and change every aspect of the relationship. The emotional bond is the main target of change. Thus, we have tended to look at the ways changes in conflict patterns, communication, and now intimacy affect the emotional bond.

Note

1 www.hopecouples.com/video-training-series

References

Arriaga, X. B., Kumashiro, M., Simpson, J. A., & Overall, N. C. (2018). Revising working models across time: Relationship situations that enhance attachment security. *Personality and Social Psychology Review, 22*(1), 71–96. https://doi.org/10.1177/1088868317705257

Chapman, G. (1992). *The Five Love Languages: How to Express Heartfelt Commitment to your Mate.* Northfield Publishing.

Chapman, G. (2023). *Love Languages. Five Love Languages.* Retrieved July 2023, from https://5lovelanguages.com/

Halpern, J. (2023, January 18). *Deep Cover: Never Seen Again.* Season 3 [Podcast]. Pushkin Industries. https://www.pushkin.fm/podcasts/deep-cover

Finkel, E. J., Rusbult, C. E., Kumashiro, M., & Hannon, P. A. (2002). Dealing with betrayal in close relationships: Does commitment promote forgiveness? *Journal of Personality and Social Psychology, 82,* 956–974.

Gottman, J. M., & Gottman, J. S. (2023). The Gottman method couple therapy. In J. L. Lebow & D. K. Snyder (Eds.), *Clinical Handbook of Couple Therapy, 6th ed.* (pp. 362–386). Guilford Press.

Johnson, D. W., & Johnson, R. T. (2006). New developments in social interdependence theory. *Genetic, Social and General Psychology Monographs, 13,* 285–358.

Karantzas, G. (2023, March 3). Is there science behind the five love languages? *Greater Good Magazine.* Retrieved July 20, 2023, from https://greatergood.berkeley.edu/article/item/is_there_science_behind_the_five_love_languages

Kelley, H. H., & Thibaut, J. (1978). *Interpersonal Relations: A Theory of Interdependence.* Wiley.

Le, B., & Agnew, C. R. (2003). Commitment and its theorized determinants: A meta-analysis of the investment model. *Personal Relationships, 10,* 37–57.

Ripley, J. S., & Worthington, E. L., Jr. (2014). *Couple Therapy: A New Hope-Focused Approach.* InterVarsity Press.

Rusbult, C. E. (1980). Commitment and satisfaction in romantic associations: A test of the investment model. *Journal of Experimental Social Psychology, 16,* 172–186.

Schaefer, M. T., & Olson, D. H. (1981). Assessing intimacy: The Pair Inventory. *Journal of Marital and Family Therapy,* 7(1), 47–60. https://onlinelibrary.wiley.com/doi/10.1111/j.1752-0606.1981.tb01351.x.

Sternberg, R. J. (1986). A Triangular Theory of Love. *Psychological Review, 93*(2), 119–135. https://doi.org/10.1037/0033-295X.93.2.119

16 Encouraging Deep Emotional Sharing

Help Partners Share Positive and Negative Emotions

Problem: Sharing emotions can be a point of weakness for couples.
Solution: Create experiences of share emotional experience.

One hot day in May, I (Jen) was feeling overwhelmed. I value my career and have experienced a sense of purpose in my work. I'm kind of a couple-therapy nerd, which you might have guessed from reading this book!

I even feel proud of using interpersonal skills learned as a couple therapist to address issues in university life. But I had a problem. Someone was thwarting my work plans and had the power to hurt me. Coworkers that I valued were divided by gossip. It surprised and shocked me. For those not in academia, the April–May time is the most stressful of the year. Graduation looms. End-of-semester, with its grading and exams, lurks. Letters for internships and jobs burden. The demands, as always, are high. But then, this shocking division threatened me.

On this day, I read a particularly harsh email, slammed the screen shut, and burst outside. My husband, Jeff, was in the front yard replanting our (excessively frustrating) grass for the third time. He had wanted me to help him with it. That had not happened. He was not happy with me. Through tears, I shared what happened in the email. He dropped his rake and hugged me for about five minutes, standing in the muddy, grassless yard. I'll never forget that moment of shared positive and negative experience. I was making a desperate bid to him for support amid my fear after I had left him without my support for his task. His hug was an act of undeserved grace. Marriages are built on shared experiences like this.

Even that shared negative experience was valued. His warm support in hugging a struggling spouse sent my feelings of bondedness through the clouds, even though at the moment I wasn't thinking about emotional

DOI: 10.4324/9781003009382-19

bonding at all. There was in the moment merely a sense that my struggle was shared.

Types of Intimacy

As we mentioned in the previous chapter, there are different types of intimacy. Let's get into each a bit deeper.

Emotional intimacy

Emotional intimacy is the perception of being close to the partner. It involves feelings of vulnerability and trust (which presumes that the partner is trustworthy and protective of one's autonomy). Emotional intimacy involves the willingness to share personal feelings, thoughts, and values within mutual sharing. Emotional intimacy makes us feel validated because someone believes we are important and meaningful. We feel that we make a difference.

Emotional sharing is dependent on emotional intimacy. If we do not believe that the partner values us and will protect our autonomy, we are unlikely to share anything that makes us vulnerable or requires trust. There will be an unconscious and implicit calculus in which we weigh the likely benefits of sharing vulnerabilities against the potential risks that we will be betrayed, devalued, or treated as someone who does not have as much worth. But such opportunities to share emotionally won't spontaneously appear. We need to make time for them (see Intervention 16-1).

Intervention 16-1 Romantic Dates and Special Times to Enhance Emotional Intimacy

During assessment, find out how couples have enhanced their romance in the past.

When you deal with intimacy, ask them to find a time to do something that can increase their emotional intimacy. Solicit their agreement not to fight or to hurt each other during that time. Have them make specific plans, set a time, and work out the details.

Follow up on this in the next session and process what did and did not work.

Ideally, having dates can pair good experiences like a new and exciting restaurant, the latest romcom or adventure movie, a moving play, a concert, or a mutually enjoyable sporting event. Couples can take hikes together, sit at a park, or go on a long drive. People don't have to go places and spend money to have such special times. They can watch a DVD or streamed movie at home, read aloud, listen to a podcast or audiobook, play games, or schedule time for sex. Sometimes, couples with children might get the kids down and then have a special meal (lobster and steak by candlelight), leave the dishes, and lock the bedroom door. Then, they can enjoy whatever goes on behind that locked door. Some couples plan time with mutual friends, their religious community, or spiritual practices as set aside time together. Dates can even become "super-dates," especially near the end of couple therapy. The superdate might be a weekend away or a vacation with just the two of them.

Romantic dates are actually comprehensive interventions, and they work well after the couple has moved past conflict and communication interventions somewhat successfully. They ask the partners to engage in emotional regulation, to communicate positively, and to enjoy romance.

Sexual intimacy

And speaking of locked bedroom doors. . . Sexual intimacy is important because it is exclusive with the partner.

Therapists should be humble when doing sexual interventions and not take on more than the couple can do. Therapists who provide sex therapy should have license-appropriate training and practice within their competency. If the couple therapist does not have such training, pursuing such specialty training is important so that they can counsel couples in sex therapy to supplement couple therapy.

If the therapist is early in career or does not have such specialty training, then couples with sexual disorders, disgust, or fear responses to sexual experiences often require a consult or referral to a specialist. Even if one has specialty training, if there are sexual problems, an appointment with a physician is usually recommended to rule out the possibility of physical causes. Therapists should be aware of and investigate whether medications or medical conditions of either partner might affect sexual functioning.

Therapists who intervene to help with sexual intimacy might approach these interventions with open communication. A decision is needed about whether sexual problems or non-sexual couple problems is primary and where treatment will focus. If sexual problems seem to be a result of other problems, low-intensity sex therapy can be tried, but if it doesn't seem to improve things within a few weeks, then a referral to specialized care or a shift in treatment goals may be needed. If you provide couple therapy involving uncomplicated sexual problems, you might provide at least three things—education, dialogue, and coaching (see Intervention 16-2).

Intervention 16-2 Three Ways to Enhance Sexual Intimacy

This intervention involves an adaptation of Ripley and Worthington (2014), BOND intervention 19-15 Improving Sexual Intimacy. Simple sensate-focus interventions may be used as homework for couples with uncomplicated poor sexual intimacy.[1]

1 **Education**. Many couples can benefit from education on what is considered normal and healthy. Younger couples, couples from sexually silent and conservative backgrounds, and those with little sexual experience often need more education. Some experience sexual problems because they lack information.
2 **Dialogue**. For couples who do not openly discuss their sexual lives, conversation is often helpful. Often, it must begin during a therapy session. Sometimes, unwillingness to discuss sex—from shyness or belief that one knows all about sex—complicates finding how to experience a satisfying sexual relationship. A therapist can help partners openly discuss their sexual needs, preferences, and desires.
3 **Coaching**. Some simple sexual therapy techniques, such as sensate focus, should be in the repertoire of most couple therapists. Sensate focus is aimed at giving and receiving pleasure rather than orgasms. Removing the goal of bringing one's partner or oneself to orgasm removes some pressure from sexual intimacy. Sensate focus times increase slowly from non-genital to genital touching and caressing. After a few weeks of practicing this several times a week, most couples are ready for sexual intercourse and orgasm.

Intellectual and recreational intimacy

Couples don't have to be "eggheads" to enjoy intellectual intimacy or "jocks" to enjoy recreational intimacy. Many couples create and maintain a bond around shared interests. A couple I (Ev) know has an extreme love of all things Star Wars, even to the point of having a fun light saber battle-dance at their wedding! They plan vacations that include Star Wars Comicon events. This shared interest in a subject matter is a kind of intellectual intimacy (and occasional recreational intimacy) that a therapist can encourage and promote. Some couples get caught in their negative cycle of relationship decline and drop common interests that they once might have enjoyed. Help partners find ways to increase intellectual and recreational intimacy (see Intervention 16-3).

Intervention 16-3 Intellectual and Recreational Intimacy

Have couples share their intellectual and reactional interests to find new avenues to improve intimacy. Sometimes, the individual interests of one partner are willing to be tried or engaged in by the other partner to increase intimacy. This intervention is especially good for couples that need to "start slow" building intimacy due to fears of more vulnerable types of intimacy.

Spiritual intimacy

Partners are connected spiritually. Sometimes, this is a shared religious spirituality. At other times, it is an alignment of values, dreams, hopes, and goals for their lives and their relationship. Emotional, sexual, intellectual, and recreational intimacy are important, as are spiritual intimacy. A classic relationship development theory (Murstein, 1970) suggested that relationships formed in stages. The first was attraction through stimuli. The second, exploration of values, which is where most spiritual intimacy is built. The third, working out roles about how to act with each other in different situations. Partners who could not find enough common ground and mutual connection at each previous stage rarely moved to the next stage. Mature couples kept paying attention to stimuli, values, and roles.

Most couples who come to couple therapy have not spent time keeping up with their partner's continually evolving interests, values, dreams, and hopes—the spiritual part of the values connection. So, often, it is helpful to reconnect spiritually. That begins with reconsidering their spirituality. Here's a classic movie that can stimulate relationship dialogue for mature couples (see Intervention 16-4).

Intervention 16-4 Prompt Spiritual and Romantic Reflection

In the classic movie *Don Juan DeMarco*, Johnny Depp plays a paranoid patient, John Arnold DeMarco, who's delusion is believing he is Don Juan. Marlon Brando plays his burned-out psychiatrist, Dr. Jack Mickler, who is retiring in ten days. As luck would have it, or good script writing, Don Juan is on a ten-day commitment. So, Dr. Mickler takes on Don Juan as his final patient. Mickler discovers in Don Juan's approach to life, the transformative truth of finding beauty in all people. He discovers that his love life with wife Marilyn (Faye Dunaway's character) has become dry and brittle. But he seeks out Marilyn's inner beauty. In a great scene, Mickler tells Marilyn, "I need to know all about you. . . . I want to know what your hopes and dreams are. I got lost along the way when I was thinking about myself." Marilyn simultaneously laughs and cries. Biting her knuckle, she says, "I thought you'd never ask."

If you assign this movie as homework, you might provide some prompts to help partners reconsider their lives together spiritually.

1 What are your hopes for the future? How does your faith/ spirituality inform those hopes?
2 How can you help your partner reach their hopes and dreams?
3 What could you do tomorrow—no matter how small—to move you along your way?

Depending on their faith perspective, some additional questions might be appropriate for religious couples.

1 What is the time in your life when you were closest to God? What happened?
2 Talk about a time when you experienced God's love or grace.
3 What is God doing in your life right now?
4 What role does sacrifice play in motivating your actions toward your partner?
5 How do your religious beliefs, values, and practices fit with your relationship?

We recommend all couples be assessed for spirituality (see Intervention 16-5). Knowing couples' spiritual connection (and for religious couples, religious connection) is important for good therapy, just like being aware of other aspects of diversity. If the therapist does not feel comfortable or competent working with religious, faithful, or spiritual couples, referral to their spiritual leader on practices or traditions that might help build spiritual intimacy.

Intervention 16-5 Assessing Spirituality with Couples

Four simple assessment questions can help understand if spirituality might be "on the table" to play a role in treatment.

1 What is your *identity* regarding religion, faith, or spirituality (R/F/S)? We have found it important to use all three of these terms because they can mean different things to different people.
2 How *prominent* is R/F/S in your life as a couple/family? This open question allows partners to share the importance (if any) of this aspect of life.
3 What *role* (if any) might R/F/S play in the problems you are facing? It might be hurtful or helpful. Religion is often like the topics of sex, money, or health. Many people will not volunteer this information because they believe you may not be interested or the topic might not be okay for therapy.
4 Do you wish R/F/S to be *included* in your therapy, and if so, how?

For couples who pray, Frank Fincham of Florida State University and Steve Beach of the University of Georgia found a power intervention for couples religiously committed to praying for each other. But this was not a "Please, God, change this person into someone easier to live with" type of prayer. Instead, it was a supportive prayer for the partner. We offer a prayer intervention idea (Intervention 16-6) for therapists looking to incorporate this with couples and families.

Intervention 16-6 Couple Prayer

Practically all religions, and even some agnostic people, engage in prayer. Therapists don't have to be religious to recommend prayer for couples who value it.

1 When introducing this, couch it generally as a way some partners have found to connect with their partner spiritually, even in couple therapy.
2 If the couple is open to prayer, ask what kinds of prayers they typically pray.
3 Ask whether prayers of blessing for each other might fit into their Couple Improvement Plan.

4 If so, the therapist tells them that quite a lot of research supports benefits of praying a warm and supportive prayer for the partner. (Prayers like, "Please fix my partner's horrible personality" are not helpful.)
5 Ask whether partners want to plan specifically when they will pray for the partner and help them make a specific plan. They might include it on their Couple Improvement Plan (Intervention 9-4; Figure 9-1).
6 In subsequent sessions, ask how this is going.

Ruptures in the Therapeutic Alliance

Dealing with religion can be a high-risk–high-reward venture. We don't always know the hidden landmines in religious partners' backgrounds, including whether they view religion the same way. Even couples who profess a strong commitment to religion might balk at using religion in couple therapy, even with a similarly religious therapist. They might balk because they might have experiences where friends or religious leaders have spiritualized advice to them, and they have come to discount that. Or they might balk if a therapist appears not knowledgeable about the religious subculture, so they view this as religious manipulation. On the other hand, some couples who are highly religiously engaged might interpret the introduction of religious considerations as a strong alliance fortifier with their therapist. Therapists are then advised to assess carefully and understand the clients, so that ruptures in the therapeutic alliance are not introduced needlessly.

So, what if a rupture in therapeutic intimacy occurs? As we likely know, and might have experienced ourselves with medical providers or professors, a rupture in the therapeutic alliance is a deterioration of the therapeutic relationship. It usually arises from disagreements about treatment goals or tasks to meet those goals or a conflict in personality styles. It also can result from emotional disconnection from irritation or frustration on the part of one or both partners or the therapist. Ruptures are related to worse therapeutic outcomes (Eubanks et al., 2018).

Therapists must try to process ruptures quickly (see Intervention 16-7). Recent research shows that it is not therapeutic ruptures per se that damage outcomes in therapy, but either reluctance of the therapist to seek to repair them or a botched repair effort characterized by failure to take appropriate responsibility or defensiveness (Eubanks et al., 2018). In this way, how you seek to repair breeches in emotional intimacy in therapy can be a role model of what partners need to be able to do: To illuminate defensive places of pain and process hurts and conflicts with empathy and understanding.

Intervention 16-7 Process Ruptures in the Therapeutic Alliance

First, apologize sincerely and thoroughly. Without excuse or defensiveness. Empathize with the pain you seem to have caused. Seek to make amends if appropriate.

Then, try to find what led to the rupture so you can avoid it in the future. Address and understand what underlying value might be threatened. That, in itself, can be rich therapeutic material.

Conclusion

Continually seek to help couples maintain, grow, and repair (if damaged) their emotional bond. Emotional sharing is an excellent way to do that, and there are many avenues to promoting emotional sharing.

Note

1 For further reading, see *Principles and Practice of Sex Therapy* by Sandra Leiblum, Guilford Press or *Enhancing Sexuality: A Problem Solving Approach to Treating Dysfunction*, by John Wincze, Oxford University Press.

References

Eubanks, C. F., Muran, J. C., & Safran, J. D. (2018). Alliance rupture repair: A meta-analysis. *Psychotherapy, 55*(4), 508–519. https://doi.org/10.1037/pst0000185. PMID: 30335462.

Leiblum, S. Risa., & Rosen, R. (2000). *Principles and Practice of Sex Therapy* (Third edition). Guilford Press.

Murstein, B. I. (1970). Stimulus value role: A theory of marital choice. *Journal of Marriage and the Family, 32*, 465–481.

Ripley, J. S., & Worthington, E. L., Jr. (2014). *Couple Therapy: A New Hope-Focused Approach*. Downers Grove, IL: InterVarsity Press.

Wincze, J. P. (2009). *Enhancing Sexuality: A Problem-Solving Approach toTtreating Dysfunction—Ttherapist Guide* (2nd ed.). Oxford University Press.

17 Balancing Intimacy and Closeness with Co-Action and Alone-Time

Find the Right Mix for Each Couple

Problem:	Intimacy requires balancing co-action and distancing across the developmental lifespan.
Solution:	Illuminate the co-action and distancing process for the couple to make intentional choices.

In the 1980s, pop psychology seemed to be obsessed with mid-life crises. If you read the work of Daniel Levinson (1978), you would believe that having a midlife crisis between ages 40 and 50 is normal. By 2004, that notion was discredited (Lachman, 2004). Clearly, though, some people did struggle with transitions. Worthington (1987) suggested that transitions happened in some couples' relationships. It was well established from cross-sectional research that average couple satisfaction changed predictably with life stage. So, what happens as couples move from stage to stage.

Changes in Couple Satisfaction with Life Stage

Years of research on heterosexual couples has shown that couple satisfaction (which is strongly related to the closeness of emotional bonding) is usually high in the early-married phase, declines at about six months (when the "honeymoon phase" is done), is lower at the birth of the first child, and declines with every child after the first. Some have called the birth of the first child a relationship "crisis" that might be even more stressful for cohabiting couples than for married couples.

Couple satisfaction is lower when the first child enters school, and is even lower as children pass through adolescence. Mark Twain had no love for children. He was reported to have said that when a child was born, they should be put in a barrel and fed through a knothole. When they reach adolescence, plug up the knothole, he advised. Certainly, on average,

DOI: 10.4324/9781003009382-20

couple satisfaction is lowest for men when children are adolescents and just as low for women.

When children begin to leave home, men experienced a surge of renewed satisfaction in the couple relationship. But for women, the children's launching was the pits—even lower couple satisfaction than when children were adolescents.

Once adjusting to all kids out of the house, though, both men and women partners recover in couple satisfaction to their early-married levels. They maintain high couple satisfaction after retiring.

Transition Theory

Could we predict which couples did and didn't have different struggles during transitions between these "stages?" Ev (Worthington, 1987) put forth a therapy-friendly theory that suggested whether couples were likely to experience a crisis during a life transition and, if so, what kind of crisis. The predicted response depended on three factors.

Disruption in intimacy–co-action–distancing and time schedules

The first factor was whether the transition caused disruption to the balance of intimacy, co-action, and distancing. Partners manage their desired intimacy–co-action–distance balance through the activities they choose, which boils down to how they spend time. Choice of career and partner significantly influences how they balance the three. A person who needs a lot of alone-time might choose a career as a writer or bookkeeper. A person who needs a lot of co-action might go into sales, which provides many interactions but little intimate sharing. A person who needs a lot of intimacy might choose to be a counselor, teacher, or a hands-on provider in a social service organization. Similarly, people choose partners because they spend time using similar patterns. For example, a person who needs a lot of intimacy will typically be drawn to a partner who also requires a lot of intimacy. This is similar with those who need mostly co-action or distancing.

Most of our time is spent in career and family relationships, so those two choices become the bedrock of happiness in managing the intimacy–co-action–distancing balance. Transitions force a rearrangement of time schedules. For example, the transition to parenthood (Roudi et al., 2013) might result in a woman who is at work less and is home more often with the child. If the woman had been working at a career not involving a lot of adult–adult interaction (say, copywriting, mostly at home), then the transition would not likely disturb her intimacy–co-action–distancing balance. She will sail through the transition going, "What's the big deal?" But suppose she had been a counselor who was used to six hours of intimate conversation helping emotionally troubled adults. After the birth, she is suddenly staying at home alone with a baby at least until her mate gets home. In that case, she might be starved for adult intimate conversation, and she counts on him taking up the slack. He will suddenly feel pressure to give much closer attention to intimate interactions with his mate. So, he will have to readjust his time commitments. Those partners will have large disruptions that might take months—or longer—to sort out.

Decisions that they disagree on initially

The second factor predicting whether a couple might have a crisis during transition is the number of new transition-related decisions they disagree about initially. Each new life transition brings things that must be decided. And, upbringing, other experiences including education, or life philosophy, can determine whether they differ on more or less decisions. If they agree on most immediately, the transition will be conflict-lite. But if they disagree about many issues, they will have many disputes to settle, and the transition will be rocky.

Presence of an active power struggle

A power struggle is essentially a struggle over who has the say about an issue. If partners are already in active power struggles, any tensions over the use of time or any disagreements will promote emotional arguments. If partners are not in a power struggle, they will face time adjustments and decisions with more equanimity.

By definition, attending couple therapy implies that a couple is facing disruption in their relationship. Their activities are unsettled. They don't agree on many crucial decisions. They are probably in an active power struggle. Their relationship is in chaos. Of course, some couples come to couple therapy because they are bored and dissatisfied. After all, they are not happy and want to change. But those are much fewer, at least in our experience. So, intimacy problems will generally require rebalancing intimacy–co-action–distancing. So how can you as therapist help?

We consider two scenarios. In the first, partners have come to the point that they want to create new bonding experiences. This is likely if (1) the couple is not heavily invested in a power struggle, (2) if the therapy work on conflict resolution and communication have gone very well, or (3) if the partners came initially more for enrichment than for therapy. In the second scenario, patterns are locked in. The emotional distancer–pursuer pattern is not the only way patterns get locked in, but it is a quintessential example. We leave it to you to generalize to other locked-in patterns.

Creating New Bonding Experiences

Creating a bonding day

The initial part of this intervention is an attempt to help couples practice more intimacy on a particular day (see Intervention 17-1). It is adapted from Fulgieri (2022, pp. 4–5; a day of love). Fulgieri's book of activities for couples is aimed at relationship enrichment for mass-market couples, not for therapy. Its basic assumption is that if partners understand what the other wants, they will try to do it. This is not usually the case when patterns of intimacy and communication are locked in. We discuss how to use the intervention, but we adapt the second part of the intervention, which teaches (by example) how inserting more intimacy into the relationship must come at the cost of replacing other activities.

Intervention 17-1 Bonding Day Activity

1. Each partner writes an ideal daily schedule, listing activities for alone-time, co-action, and intimacy.
2. Add one or two activities you would like to do with your partner and one or two you would like to do for your partner.
3. Examine the schedule and see what would change if you did the new activities. Especially watch for preferences in intimacy, co-action, and distancing (or you might use the term autonomy with couples as it has less negative connotations).
4. Ask the couple to pick a day to carry out the ideal bonding day.
5. As you process this with the couple, ask specifically about what they had to change and give up to make a more intimate day. See if you can draw out the point that life is a balance of intimacy–co-action–distancing and thus, making changes needs to be done with awareness of what else is affected.

Partners create a "user-friendly manual to love me"

Again, this is adapted from Fulgieri (2022, pp. 6–7; manual for loving me). In Intervention 17-2, partners create a "user-friendly manual" specifying what they believe would communicate love and intimacy. We again adapt this to help partners consider what must be foregone if the new actions are taken.

Intervention 17-2 A User-friendly Manual to Love Me

1 Have both partners create a "user-friendly" manual to help the other partner care for them. This identifies:

   i things they regularly need;
   ii things they need specifically from their partner;
   iii cautions to the partner about things they are particularly sensitive to.

2 Each partner gives their manual to the partner to read.
3 Discuss in session the major points, looking for things that are not provided at present and asking whether those could be provided in the future.
4 Importantly, ask what would be given up if the new actions are begun.
5 See if partners are willing to put this into action for a week and process the outcomes in the next session.

For example, a woman highlighted identify affirmation, respect, being listened to, time to talk about things that matter, and time to cuddle intimately (without sex) as five things she needs. She also suggested that before the partner initiates any of these, a direct question, "Is this a good time to . . ." would be appreciated because it respects her wishes and time. As partners discussed these, they found that affirmation, respect, and the prefacing with "Is this a good time to . . ." were all agreeable suggestions that require little time to enact, even though they require energy and attention to remember to do. However, making time to talk more than they did, spend time in non-sexual cuddling, and simply spending more time together all required deciding what each partner had to give up to make time for those activities. That discussion was difficult and allowed them to put their conflict-resolution and communication lessons into practice so they could work out a way to enact these changes.

Couples Who Are Locked into Patterns by Power Struggles

Interventions 17-3, 17-4, and 17-5 are aimed at couples who have entrenched patterns of intimacy–co-action–distancing and communication. One example of such an entrenched pattern is the emotional distancer–pursuer dynamic (Guerin et al., 1996). For example, Sam and Roni are madly in love and enjoy being together most of the time. Yet lately, they find they have had arguments. After a particularly rough fight, Roni complained,

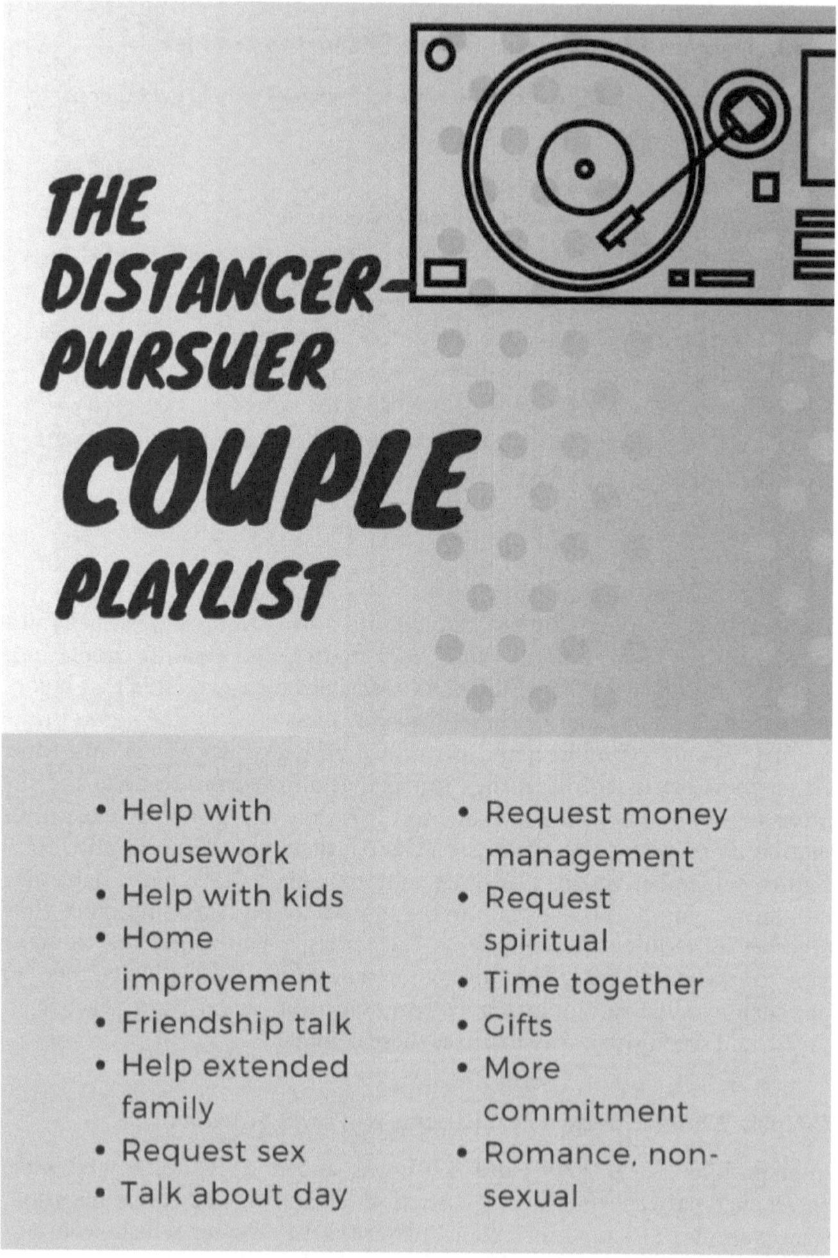

Figure 17-1 The Distancer–Pursuer Couple Playlist. Topics that Trigger the Pattern of Requesting Interaction Followed by Withdrawal Followed by Elevated Intensity of Requests, etc.

"Sam just stares at screens with the phone all the time. It's like I'm not even here. When I ask for conversation or time together, I get nothing." The therapist turns to Sam, who responds, "We've been together for a while. My business requires me to post on social media all the time, and I have to concentrate. I don't have the time I used to."

Distancer–pursuer patterns happen in almost every relationship. However, in healthy relationships, the roles of distancer and pursuer are more flexible and less extreme. As relationships deteriorate, roles solidify and get more hostile. Fears and conflicts aren't processed. Ruminations rule the roost for couples like Sam and Roni.

Calling out the pattern

The most straightforward intervention for this process is to illuminate the process for the couple and have them reflect on it. Sometimes that even works. Sometimes. But it's worth a try (see Intervention 17-3). The distancer–pursuer playlist (Figure 17-1) provides an example.

This intervention uses the metaphor of a "playlist" to help couples identify patterns they use so often that they get old and boring. Comedian John Mulaney tells how he played a prank by playing Tom Jones's song "What's New Pussycat?" 21 times on a jukebox. The trapped diners were completely insane and ready to murder him. The bit is called "Salt and Pepper Diner." It can be found with a Google search. (Warning: the content is pretty "salty.") The point of the joke is that even great ideas get old, especially if they're not the best idea. And this distancer–pursuer pattern is not the best idea.

Couples can explore which topics trigger their distancer–pursuer patterns. These can include becoming emotionally blocked, defensiveness, criticism, inducing guilt, making demands instead of requests, using coercion, using hostility or verbal aggression, putting down the other person, and whining or complaining.

Intervention 17-3 Distancer–Pursuer Playlist

After the therapist has observed the pattern of a request by the pursuer being met with withdrawal and non-response by the distancer followed by escalation of the intensity of the request (soon-to-be demand), and then of the response (or non-response), the therapist suggests that he or she has seen an interaction repeat a few times. The therapist names the sequence of actions. The next time this is observed, the therapist suggests that "This *might* be a pattern with you both." The next time, "I'm seeing this pattern repeat."

Suggest that this is like a playlist of different songs in which the same type repeat.

Enlist the partners in identifying topics that trigger this pattern (aka songs on the distancer–pursuer playlist). Write up the playlist (see Figure 17-1).

Coach partners to recognize when they are playing a song on the playlist. Show them how to ask whether they want to change the song by breaking the pattern.

Plan alternative responses that break up the pattern without always giving in to the pursuer or to the distancer. This might be turn-taking or partners might come up with a different solution that works for them.

Accepting the pattern

One of the best theoretical contributions of integrative behavioral couple therapy (ICBT; Christensen et al., 2020) is that no couple can change every process that is not healthy for their relationship. Thus, there are just things they must decide to accept and move on. Coupled with that insight, ICBT found that processes of influence can become unhealthy cyclical patterns of conflict that are mutually destructive (see Intervention 17-4). We've also called these power struggles. Acceptance then takes the form of lowering attempts to over-influence the partner and reasonably accepting some influence from the partner. This solution depends on realizing that giving up a little influence is less noxious than engaging in a noxious ongoing power struggle.

Intervention 17-4 Influencing Well and Accepting Influence

This is one way to deal with the emotional distancer–pursuer pattern. The pursuer in this intervention is likely over-influencing the partner with poor, negative, and frequent tactics to get more closeness. Ask pursuers if they want to get what they need without damaging the relationship.

Help them empathize with the distancing partner's pain. The distancer is often flooded with negative emotions and fear of failing their partner. This sometimes surprises the pursuing partner (and novice therapist) because the distancer appears cool and unaffected. Yet, the distancer's withdrawal is often a poor attempt at managing strong negative emotions, not rejection of intimacy. Fear is easier to empathize with than an attribution of rejection. Show the pursuer more effective, soft, and thoughtful ways to make requests.

Distancers are often persuaded to distance less if they can empathize with the underlying needs of the pursuing partner. Pursuers are often afraid of rejection and insecure about whether they are loved (or sometimes that they are worthy of love). Coach distancers to seek to meet the pursuer's needs for reassurance directly. Perhaps coach them to offer to help but, if now is not a good time, to say explicitly when will be a good time, and then be sure to follow through.

If the couple continues stubborn distancer–pursuer patterns, dig deeper into childhood patterns or emotional losses and traumas that might fuel the pattern. Sometimes, people have made "inner vows" to "never be hurt like that again" in such a way they will engage in desperate tactics that undermine all relationships. Some partners also need distress-tolerance skill-building, such as those found in dialectical behavior therapy (McKay et al., 2019) approach paired with couple interventions.

Dealing with the power struggle

You can't resolve a power struggle if it exists. But, as you work with the couple, here are three paths (see Intervention 17-5) you might guide them toward to help them arrive at workable solutions.

Intervention 17-5 Healthy Paths to Intimacy and Independence

Help them understand each other better. We all need both intimacy and independence. The skilled therapist calmly and confidently responds, saying, "Ah, the great couple problem: You are not the same person and don't exist as personal assistants for the other. Partners become better, more mature, and kind if they learn how to live in the ever-changing flow of needs for companionship vs. autonomy. Tell me, [time-alone partner], what do you need from your partner regarding companionship, affection, input, and care for you? And for you, [need-people partner], when do you also need to make your own choices, be trusted to operate yourself without checking in, and have some quiet moments alone?"

It's not a zero-sum game. The partners seem to be assuming that they are the only provider of social interaction or respecter of alone-time. So, they can be approached directly with guidance something like this: "Next, let's talk about how to get needs met across all parts of life. Can you each talk about how your needs for intimacy and independence are met outside of your relationship?" This is the more unstructured approach.

Or, in a more structured approach you could give each a sheet of paper. Have them create two columns, one for each need. On the intimacy side, discuss ways they get closeness needs met throughout other aspects of life besides their couple relationship. Perhaps the pursuer can create more intimacy time with same-sex friends or family or those who they are now acquaintances with but would like to know better. Perhaps the distancer can reduce non-essential social interaction to feel more able to be more social with the partner. Similarly for independence or aloneness. Can the pursuer create more intimacy and therefore cherish the aloneness when with the partner? Can the distancer create more distance in non-partner interactions so that not as much aloneness is needed with the partner?

Coach partners to accept what they cannot change. This was covered in Intervention 17-4.

Conclusion

One of the overlooked aspects of managing intimacy needs is how partners use their 24 hours of each day. This is a practical focus for managing intimacy, but very effective.

References

Christensen, A., Doss, B. D., & Jacobson, N. S. (2020). *Integrative Behavioral Couple Therapy: A Therapist's Guide to Creating Acceptance and Change (2nd ed)*. W. W. Norton.

Fulgieri, M. (2022). *Couple Therapy Activity Book: 65 Creative Activities to Improve*

Communication and Strengthen your Relationship. Rockridge Press.

Guerin, P. J., Jr., Fogarty, T. F., Fay, L. F., & Kautto, J. G. (1996). *Working with Relationship Triangles: One-Two-Three of Psychotherapy*. Guilford Press.

Lachman, M. (2004). Development in mid-life. *Annual Review of Psychology, 55*, 305–331.
Levinson, D. (1978). *The Seasons of a Man's Life*. Ballentine Books.
McKay, M., Wood, J. C. & Brantley, J. (2019) *The Dialectical Behavior Therapy skills workbook: Practical DBT exercises for learning mindfulness, interpersonal effectiveness, emotion regulation, and distress tolerance*. New Harbinger Publications.
Roudi, N. R., Schumm, W. R., & Britt, S. L. (2013). *Transition to Parenthood*. Springer.
Worthington, E. L., Jr. (1987). Treatment of families during life transitions: Matching treatment to family response. *Family Process, 26*, 295–308.

18 Discerning Attachment Styles and Emotional Bonds

Find Effects of Early Relationships and of Adult Ones

Problem:	Attachment styles need to be understood and accommodated.
Solution:	Create experiences with couples that clarify attachment-driven processes and create new healing experiences.

Research on couples counseling has repeatedly shown that one key to relationship change is improving the adult attachments of partners (Muetzefeld et al., 2021). Adult attachment is the secure emotional connection that a person feels exists between the partners (Shaver & Mikulincer, 2010). Couples who are secure in their adult attachment are not avoidant or anxious about their relationship. They have faith in their relationship. They have faith in each other as a safe, secure base for relating. Secure partners can get their needs met either through their relationship (interdependent) or on their own (independent). They are comfortable with being known and intimately knowing others, which frees them to love and work.

How Attachment Styles Affect (and Don't Affect) Emotional Bonds

Attachment styles are generally organized into four typologies (Shaver & Mikulincer, 2010), which are the interplay of two interpersonal traits on bell curves: anxiety and avoidance. People with:

- Anxious-preoccupied attachment style (15% of the population) worry, have emotional hunger for ideal love, tend to cling if needs aren't met, have high anxiety, and have low avoidance.

DOI: 10.4324/9781003009382-21

- Avoidant attachment style (23%) are distant, independent, tend to process their needs and emotions without personal interaction, shut down when threatened, have low anxiety, and have high avoidance.
- Disorganized attachment style (1–5%) vacillate between a desperate need for the attachment figure and pushing them away, have unpredictable moods, have both high anxiety and avoidance.
- Secure attachment style (62%) have both low anxiety and avoidance, form connections easily, have faith in their relationships, are calm when together but comfortable asking for help or comfort.

One of the more curious parts of couple therapy is that both partners may have relatively good adult attachment styles. Still, circumstances and the couple's dynamics can keep them in a weak, damaged, or even undeveloped emotional bond within the specific couple relationship.

Attachment models like the security enhancement model (Arriaga et al., 2018) have support. It is more probable for insecure partners to create unhealthy couple bonds, but *anyone* can get caught in a negative relational loop. Couples can enact unhealthy relational patterns, even with secure interpersonal styles. Extreme stress, trauma, illness, disability, mental disorders, discrimination, spiritual crisis, grief, loss, and scarcity can all affect couples' ability to cope as a team.

Secure partners who experience a disastrous relationship can sometimes find it difficult to bond with their next partner. Across a lifetime, every couple will experience some of these things and can easily get caught in a negative dynamic and ask us for help. Partners in extreme stress can often *appear* insecure for a while. Not all partners are skilled at responding to their normally secure partner suddenly having needs.

Situational influences have been recognized in research to a point where models that include factors like emotional intelligence, control in a situation, partner behaviors, relationship goals, and appraisals influence partner dynamics (Chen & Liao, 2021). We can say for certain that attachment style is not the whole story of a couple's emotional bonds.

Interventions to Strengthen Emotional Bonds through Using Attachment Styles

Strengthening emotional bonds is, in many ways, where the couple-therapy action is. By the time you work directly on emotional bonds in couple therapy, you have had to work through conflicts and communication—which strengthen bonds but do so indirectly—to earn the right to help work to repair and strengthen emotional bonds directly. Let's look at some direct interventions.

Help partners understand intergenerational influences of attachment styles using genograms

We won't re-explain the family genogram intervention because almost all marriage and family classes or books provide training in genogram interventions. If you have missed this intervention, you can find some supportive material in any family therapy text, web search, or our website, www.hopecouples.com. If partners are especially unclear about different attachment styles, brief questionnaires are available online.

One method of using genograms is to help partners understand attachment styles and to examine their current genogram pattern in light of their family history (see Intervention 18-1). Anxious or avoidant traits begin in the family of origin, and research supports neurobiological influence (Cacioppo et al., 2014). Children often repeat scripts or dynamics that shape how they think they should interact with others. Those scripts are reflected in mirror neurons, which are active when people copy others' behaviors. This biological path shapes relational behaviors rooted in early learning.

Intervention 18-1 Understand Attachment by Creating Genograms Focused on Attachment Styles

Explain what genograms are. Have partners, between sessions, construct their own genogram as far back as they can. Have them focus on the adult attachment of each partner in each relationship. Then, at the next session, discuss their perceptions of each partner's attachment style in their own relationship. Discuss how the styles might have been passed along through generations.

Theorists once proposed that attachment styles were "set" by age 5, with little change in adulthood. That is no longer believed. Adult relationships can rewire attachment styles, even neurobiologically (Fishbane, 2013). Repeated experiences of adult relationships and interpersonal traumas, such as the discovery of infidelity, can override early attachment styles (Warach & Josephs, 2021).

Partners' attachment styles in their romantic relationship

The good news is that origin is not destiny. Certainly, the attachment styles we learned and practiced through childhood and adolescence stamp us indelibly. But we usually experience adult romantic relationships after childhood is gone. We enter the first of those with our family-of-origin template. But our actual romantic relationships can override much of that template. Secure attachment from one's family of origin can be shattered by an abusive romantic partner. That can make entering into marriage or a marriage-like relationship feel like one has an anxious, avoidant, or disorganized-neglected attachment style. Similarly, a mature romantic relationship can largely heal an insecure attachment style from one's family of origin. Using Intervention 18-2, we help partners explore their adult attachment styles.

Intervention 18-2 Attachment Styles in Their Close Relationships

1 Have partners recall their primary attachment style from their family of origin.
2 Ask each to think of the one or two romantic relationships they had before their current relationship. Then, have them discuss each relationship and how it might have shifted (perhaps dramatically, perhaps more of an evolution than revolution) their adult attachment style.
3 Draw a box with the four attachment styles and have the partners note where they were when they became serious about each other romantically.
4 Have them talk about how they see themselves now.

Move from partner- to couple-thinking

If you've had partners try to identify their primary attachment styles and talk about how those might have led to the adult attachment style in their romantic relationship, then you can have them think about how the two styles can together make up a stable emotional bond (see Intervention 18-3). This is a crucial move from individual perspective (i.e., how each partner has an attachment style) to how these affect the emotional bond between them.

Intervention 18-3 Two Attachment Styles, One Emotional Bond

1 Identify attachment styles in childhood and currently. You can search for reputable online quizzes by universities where attachment labs have been ongoing, like UCLA and Cornell University.

2 Make an informative but neutral statement about the emotional bond. Reiterate that partners have already identified early and beginning-relationship and current-status-of-relationship attachment styles.
3 The important thing is how they fit together as a couple to shape their bond during positive and negative events and how resilient or brittle the bond is. Say, "Some people have such strongly influential pasts that their pasts tend to push the entire relationship. For most people, the past is not as influential."
4 Have them talk about their emotional bond in light of their and their partner's attachment styles. Let them take the lead. You can illuminate processes that may need help clarifying.

Therapy Issues in Dealing with Strengthening the Emotional Bond

Some common issues recur across couples as they deal with closeness. So, we wanted to mention three that are frequent.

It's okay to deviate from the treatment plan to repair damage to the emotional bond

Interventions can be technically beautiful. But if they are not done in love, they can be harmful. A couple had worked well in therapy up to the 12th week. This was to be the second week discussing forgiveness. They had agreed to write five apology notes to each other to read aloud in this week's session. The therapist asked about whether partners did the homework but skipped asking about their week. They both reported having written the apology notes.

> Wife: I am sorry that my criticisms have been so hurtful to your *tender* heart that is deeply sensitive to anything that is not positive and encouraging.

The "tender-hearted" husband was a special forces operative who would intimidate a bear. He was far from sensitive, and he oozed arrogance. That had been his wife's complaint from the intake. So, the sarcasm could be carved with a broadsword. The wife didn't gloat long.

> Husband: I apologize that my withdrawal into my Ham Radio hobby leaves you lonely since you don't have any friends or family here who care about you.

She didn't have any friends or family because the couple had moved to a new city just three months earlier. For his career. She was insecure about whether she was loved and even lovable.

These are the moments that try therapists' souls. The therapist knew the couple's backgrounds enough to feel the cruel jabs. He stopped that exercise and dropped back to ask, "So, let's stop here. What happened this week? Something seems to have."

Both partners had had stressful weeks punctuated by an argument. After that, they had regressed into distancing and lobbing criticisms at each other. Neither felt supported in their own struggles, so they lashed out.

The therapist made an error in not asking about the couple's week. But he saw that error and quickly aborted the homework, which likely would have yielded more hurts, and went back to seeking to repair damage done to the emotional bond.

Predict backsliding

We cannot always see that problems will occur. But sometimes we can. We have noticed a pattern that our psychodynamic friends could have warned us of decades ago. When a couple successfully bonds after a period of animosity, they often have a defensive week. One can even predict it for the couple, as in Intervention 18-4.

Intervention 18-4 Predict Backsliding to Avoid It

This therapist models predicting backsliding after an advance in session.

> "We just had a great moment here, I think. You each shared a deep-felt need and insecurity, and you each responded with care and vulnerability. I couldn't be prouder of you two.
>
> As you head out this week, if you are like many couples, you can expect to feel some fear around that vulnerability. You might feel a pull to return to old patterns and defenses. That's normal if it happens, but hopefully you can see it coming and not fall into the trap that many other couples do.
>
> How could you respond compassionately to yourself or your partner if you feel old defenses pop up?"

Ways to address defenses

If the couple is ready—if this isn't their first success but you sense they are moving toward a strong bond—you might even explore reasons for long-standing defenses attempting (poorly) to hold up weak emotional bonds. Some defenses may have begun in childhood, in an earlier relationship, in the workplace. If partners have repeated experiences of interpersonal fear and danger, their attachment style can deteriorate.

You may ask, "What do I do if the couple is *not ready* to be vulnerable to explore childhood defenses or respond compassionately to their partner's defenses?" Some version of this question is one of the most common questions I (Jen) get in supervision or when consulting on cases. Intervention 18-5 is our grab-bag of responses to defenses.

Intervention 18-5 Address Defenses against Vulnerability

When partners seem defensive and are unable to either explore their own defenses or are unable to help their partner, use whichever of these seems most appropriate.

- Be calm, curious, and compassionate. Even if partners can't yet display these traits, the therapist can model how to do it.
- Match the session's emotional valence to the couple's developmental level. The couple may not be able to emotionally bond deeply. Therapy involves joining their pain to illuminate their "next step" toward their goals. Small gains fuel larger risk-taking.
- Assess where the defenses are coming from. Is the person weighed down with severe depression? Personality disorder? Trauma reactivity? Low emotional intelligence? Do you completely understand why they feel vulnerable and need to defend themselves?
- Explore childhood contributions to the defense. Ask things like, "What would your family have done in this situation?" Curiously wonder whether they are repeating patterns learned early in life. That question at least pulls blame away from the partner toward a time before their relationship.
- Portray the defense as a problem for both partners, not one. If the defense is to withdraw, then discuss how withdrawal is self-protective but creates a problem for closeness. It's not one person's problem. It's a collective problem to solve as a team.

- Ask what the defense is trying to tell everyone. The therapist can explore what underlying fear, vulnerability, or anger may be fueling the defense. Then the therapist can put words to that defense: "Don't ask too much of me. I'll probably fail you. So, you're better off if I withdraw."
- The "monsters/demons on the boat" intervention from acceptance and commitment therapy (ACT) can be helpful when intense fears fuel defenses. The therapist helps the partner identify unsought goals and unused values due to fears. Partners work as a team to identify the voices of fear and to soothe them when trying to obtain goals despite fears. If you are unfamiliar with this intervention, you can find more about it in ACT training materials or an internet search.

Solidifying Strong Emotional Bonds Near the End of Therapy

Because of the centrality of strengthening the emotional bond, we don't believe you can pay too much attention to it. As couple therapy winds down, there are times when reinforcing gains are possible. Here are two of those times.

Renewal of vows

Couples may benefit from renewing their vows. Some cultural groups value vow-making in relationships. For others, they enter implicit contracts. Vows (or verbalizing the implicit contract) help the couple bond. We often use a vow-renewal ceremony (see Intervention 18-6) in the last session for couples whose couple therapy has gone well.

Intervention 18-6 Solidify Intimacy by Renewing Vows

As homework, ask the partners to write down their vows to each other for renewing in the upcoming session. Encourage them to talk about what is relevant to their relationship today and identify things they intend to practice over the long haul. Some couples have created an event to renew vows, like a party or gathering of friends, and included others through various social media posts.

Create a sojourner narrative (Intervention 18-7)

Instead of taking vows that focus on the future exclusively, some couples prefer to see their relationship as a journey in which they travel together for some shared purpose. This intervention allows a partner's experiences to be set within a narrative of personal growth and change. This is also a good to use late in counseling or at termination. It can also be used early in couple therapy to create goals for couple therapy.

Intervention 18-7 Solidify Intimacy by Creating a Sojourning Narrative[1]

The partners each write a narrative of their life experiences with a prospective ending that involves growth and transformation. As they discuss it in session, the therapist is scribe, writing major concepts they discuss. As partners discuss their stories, they are encouraged to gain perspective on where they have been and are going. Their narrative has three parts:

1 My journey before you,
2 Our journey together, and
3 Our future.

Other interventions that can be drawn upon are the intake (informing "My journey before you"), some other aspects of the intake and graphs of closeness, or types of love as they changed with time (informing "Our journey together"), and best hopes and dreams for counseling vision-casting for the future of the relationship (informing "Our future"). If the first two parts are addressed in session, partners can be asked to reflect on "Our future" as the therapy nears termination.

Conclusion

All of therapy is aimed indirectly or directly at creating, strengthening, maintaining, or repairing the emotional bond between partners. In the chapters in the current part of the book, we looked at directly affecting the emotional bond. In the following part, we look at repairing it through forgiving and reconciling.

Note

1 Adapted from Ripley & Worthington, 2014, BOND Intervention 19-17, Sojourning Together

References

Arriaga, X. B., Kumashiro, M., Simpson, J. A., & Overall, N. C. (2018). Revising working models across time: Relationship situations that enhance attachment security. *Personality and Social Psychology Review, 22*(1), 71–96. https://doi.org/10.1177/1088868317705257

Cacioppo, S., Zhou, H., Monteleone, G., Majka, E. A., Quinn, K., Ball, A. B., Norman, G. J., Semin, G. R. & Cacioppo, J. T. (2014). You are in sync with me: Neural correlates of interpersonal synchrony with a partner. *Neuroscience, 277*, 842–858. https://doi.org/10.1016/j.neuroscience.2014.07.051

Chen, W.-L., & Liao, W. T. (2021). Emotion regulation in close relationships: The role of individual differences and situational context. *Frontiers in Psychology, 12*, 697901–697901. https://doi.org/10.3389/fpsyg.2021.697901

Fishbane, M. D. (2013). *Loving with the Brain in Mind: Neurobiology and Couple Therapy (Norton Series on Interpersonal Neurobiology)*. W. W. Norton & Company.

Muetzelfeld, H., Megale, A., Friedlander, M. L., & Xu, M. (2021). Relations between attachment insecurity and role and outcome expectations for couple therapy. *Journal of Family Therapy, 43*(1), 64–77. https://doi-org.ezproxy.regent.edu/10.1111/1467-6427.12306

Ripley, J. S., & Worthington, E. L., Jr. (2014). *Couple Therapy: A New Hope-Focused Approach*. Downers Grove, IL: InterVarsity Press.

Shaver, P. R., & Mikulincer, M. (2010). New directions in attachment theory and research. *Journal of Social and Personal Relationships, 27*(2), 163–172. https://doi.org/10.1177/0265407509360899

Warach, B., & Josephs, L. (2021). The aftershocks of infidelity: A review of infidelity-based attachment trauma. *Sexual and Relationship Therapy, 36*(1), 68–90.

Part 4

Forgiving

19 Dealing with Hurts and Injustices

Reduce the Injustice Gap to Make Forgiveness Easier

Problem:	Offenses create an injustice gap in a couple relationship.
Solution:	Actions that reduce the injustice gap, other than forgiveness, help couples reconnect after offenses.

Ellie had a rough background. She had a history of substance abuse in her teens and early 20s after escaping a deeply neglectful home life. Life was unfair, she concluded.

Now, however, she had finally found "the one," and she and Mark had moved in together and had a tiny baby. Mark was rough, military-enlisted, often-deployed, and low in empathy. While Mark walked into the relationship with his own set of troubles, he was at least safe, quiet, non-abusive, sober, and came home every night when not deployed. Everything seemed fine. Then Ellie left.

Mark got a call from their neighbor. She was looking after their baby, and she said that she wondered when Ellie was coming back. Ellie's old friend had called with an emergency. Ellie left with him, and no one knew where she was for four days. Finally, Ellie's mother, concerned about the baby, tracked Ellie down. Ellie had had a brief affair with the old friend, used drugs again, then, the fling over, come back to Mark and the baby two weeks later. How unfair and hurtful this was to Mark!

How would you treat this couple? They have present dysfunction, recent injustices, and many past injustices that might be at the root of present struggles. It can be tempting to stop treatment with a couple like Mark and Ellie once their high-pain problem has been addressed and they seem to be reconnected. Some therapists think, "Great. We're done! Let's close up this case."

Not so fast. The relationship can quickly lose the hard-won gains if partners haven't addressed past hurts. They then have to put those past

DOI: 10.4324/9781003009382-23

injustices and hurts into perspective. Amanda Ripley (2021), in her book, *High Conflict*, says that people need to see things from the balcony, and not just retain the ground-floor perspective in which the problems developed. Only then can they commit to moving on and not have to worry that the past will bite them in the behind.

In this chapter, we describe how to deal with perceived injustices. There are many ways, and we cover alternatives to forgiving injustices in this chapter. We'll get to forgiveness in the following chapter.

The Injustice Gap

The *injustice gap* is the difference between how we would like a perceived injustice dealt with and how we currently see it. When partners interact with each other over a long period, each can perceive an injustice gap. This is just something human. We always see what we do, but we don't see everything that the other person does and we don't see struggles that the other person has at trying not to hurt us. The bottom line is that almost no couple believes that, in their relationship, perfect justice reigns. For most couples, the goal is usually a just-good-enough balance of justice.

Each partner has a perceived injustice gap. We can take it for granted that the contents and sizes of the gaps are different for each partner. When couple troubles exist, we can assume that the gaps are large. So, we want to help each person work on their injustice gap.

Many actions can lower the perceived size of a person's injustice gap. These can be soft emotional interactions, kind acts, or directly repaying for something lost or damaged. Forgiveness is one way of getting past that gap, which is often ideal for couples to deal with the accumulated hurts and injustices. However, many other ways exist to deal with the partners' injustice gaps. Those other ways are the focus of this chapter.

Justice is often portrayed as a scale. Experiencing a perceived injustice weighs down one side of the scale. If the other person does something costly and self-sacrificial—like apologizing or groveling—we think, *That's justice. It helps balance the scale.* But almost never will that one act completely balance the scales. While the weight of injustice may decrease, it usually requires more to fully restore balance. So, we expect more.

Imagine that the size of an injustice gap is like a wall that a person must overcome to move on with the relationship. Each bit of justice done knocks some height from the top of the wall. The likelihood of getting over the wall, by say, receiving another self-sacrificial act, by turning the matter over to God, or by forgiving, is inversely proportional to the size of the injustice gap. Big injustice gaps = harder to deal with. Small gaps = easier to deal with.

Some injustice gaps are HUGE. One partner has hurt the other hundreds of times. Or has betrayed the trust of the partner. Or had an affair. The injustice-gap wall feels 50 feet tall. There seems to be no way to get over it. At least, at first. When injustice gaps are HUGE, multiple efforts to whack height from the wall are usually needed to balance the scale.

Handling Hurts by Reducing the Size of the Injustice Gap

In the Chapter 20, we will feature the REACH forgiveness intervention to help people get past memories of hurts with grace and mercy. That intervention is to forgive. Many clients have had negative experiences with forgiveness or feel it is coercive, usually because they have been subjected to well-meaning people who have used forgiveness coercively. Such people are wary of it and (let's face it) perhaps prejudiced against it due to past experiences or perhaps associating forgiveness with religion when they are not personally religious.

Yet couples like Ellie and Mark have deep hurts that need to be repaired. Fortunately, forgiveness is not the only avenue to repairing hurts. And even if the person forgives, forgiveness does not have to do all the heavy lifting. Couples can and do use many strategies to deal with the injustices. In this chapter, we examine the creative repair of hurts and injustices that do not use forgiveness.

Options to Repair Relationships Besides Forgiveness

One way to organize our options for relationship repair is to place them into three categories. These are actions to promote justice, response strategies that can improve things, and psychological guidance to lower the injustice gap.

Actions to promote justice

Direct actions by the offended person and sometimes the offender can lower the offended person's sense of injustice. The offended person can:

- Offer and make (or the offended person can obtain) restitution (in some other way). Restitution is restoring losses that the offended person incurred. The key to restitution is that the losses are accurately identified and restitution is seen as fair compensation for losses incurred. Restitution can be part of making amends, a broader term that includes apologies and efforts to amend errors, mistakes, or injustices and even make up for suffering caused by the injustice. Restitution is limited to

direct compensation replacing losses incurred. Restitution can never completely make up for what was lost because it does not compensate for suffering, betrayal, etc.
- Eschew revenge. Refusing to seek revenge is not forgiving, but a decision to forgive does involve a refusal to seek revenge.
- Turn the matter over to a higher power or God for divine justice.

Either partner can:

- Bring about a more just situation. Seeing justice done could be through the justice system or informally by seeing a person get just desserts each reduce the offended person's injustice gap.
- Both partners can:
- Decide to interact trustworthily and follow though.

Response strategies to make things better

These are the adoption of a strategic way of acting regarding injustice. The offended person can:

- Tolerate the injustice. People tolerate injustice when they decide simply not to respond.
- Forbear. Forbearing is choosing to suppress all signs of upset toward the other, which, to that point, is similar to tolerating injustice. But forbearance has a reason for suppressing negative responses—it is done for harmony in the relationship or group.
- Accept. Simply accept that bad things happen and move on with life.
- Relinquish the matter to God, karma, or fate without expectation of seeing justice.

Psychological guidance to lower the injustice gap

These are attempts to recast the situation in a less unjust way. The offended partner can:

- Make different attributions about what offended: that excuse (appealing to extenuating circumstances) or justify (appealing to the notion that the person had a just right to harm or offend one) the offense.
- Reduce the intensity of negative emotions by self-soothing. Self-soothing is a great psychological tool for reining negative emotions and allowing for productive interaction. But self-soothing of one's legitimate, just feelings and moral evaluations merely to calm oneself usually miscarries justice.
- Empathize with the offender. Sometimes, that empathy can overwhelm the feelings of injustice that were experienced. Empathizing with the

offender does not change the injustice, and most people can empathize without losing objectivity in evaluating wrongdoing.
- Look honestly at one's own contributions to a hurtful situation, which sometimes can create a sense of justice. The person can see his or her contribution and might conclude that there was no net injustice. Often, though, people tend to value their suffering as worth more than the suffering they inflict. Thus, when a person concludes that there was no net injustice, it often means, in reality, the other person will believe there was a large injustice done.
- Create personal meaning out of the offense. This usually involves benefit-finding from the offense that justifies ignoring some or all of the injury from the offense.
- Use stress-management coping methods that involve problem-focused, emotion-focused, and meaning-focused coping. These action-oriented strategies don't precisely bring justice to the situation. Still, they are active (problem-focused and emotion-focused coping) or cognitive (meaning-focused coping) strategies for changing one's stressfulness associated with injustice.
- Reduce rumination through various methods, such as mindfulness, which focuses on the present. Rumination keeps the injustice fresh on people's minds, so psychological interventions that reduce rumination can reduce the perceived injustice simply because the injustice is perceived less frequently.

None of these are forgiveness, but they are generally good actions to take in response to an offense. Each reduces the size of the injustice gap, making forgiveness more likely. Some clients may need these additional ways to address hurts in their relationship. The use of several methods (of which forgiveness might be one) is highly recommended. We will illustrate several but not all of these in the remainder of the present chapter. To help you think more in terms of how you might help people by affecting the injustice gap rather than relying on specific interventions, we have organized these interventions into two groups—those that primarily affect the injustice gap by changing cognition and those that affect the injustice gap by different actions.

Cognitive Adjustment of the Injustice Gap

Some people struggle more with their thoughts and reactions to offenses than others. This may be due to their perception of the event, disposition, personality, past, or relationship dynamics. Stopping rumination and emotional floods from injustice gaps is harder for some people than others.

Get a "balcony" perspective

Sometimes it helps to get a higher, "balcony," perspective on hurtful and unjust events (Ripley, 2021). Intervention 19-1 offers a story that might help people shift their perception.

Intervention 19-1 See with Magic Eyes Fable

Ask the couple to read and reflect on the fable.

Lewis Smedes is an author and theologian who wrote a fable called "The Magic Eyes" (a Google search should find it) that reflects on a husband's hollow forgiveness for his wife's infidelity. Hollow forgiveness is when one pretends to forgive to use their right-ness to make the person feel even worse. In the story, an angel came to the husband each time he felt hatred toward his wife and dropped a small pebble in his heart, which made his heart heavy. Then the angel comes to the husband and offers the remedy for his heavy heart—to see with "magic eyes." Each time the husband replaced his vision of his wife as a betrayer with seeing his wife as a weak woman who needed him, a pebble would be removed from his heart. After initially rejecting the magic eyes, the pain was so great that he accepted the gift from the angel and slowly began to remove the pebbles from his heart.

Disposition or personality

Some types of personalities habitually create hard-to-repair offenses (Fincham et al., 2005). Toxic cognition includes negative rumination, resentment, avoidance, revenge-seeking, and blame. Partners with hostile or narcissistic personalities tend to be intolerant of offenses, making it more difficult to repair them. Personality characteristics of low agreeableness and high neuroticism (i.e., emotional reactivity) are associated with difficulty forgiving and relationship problems in general. As therapists work with various clients on forgiveness, they will want to adjust expectations and prognosis based on disposition or personality factors.

Pasts

Typically, couples with one big transgression are more likely to be able to repair the relationship than are partners with a multitude of moderate hurts, or a relationship that has escalated in divisiveness in ways that parallel Gottman's Four Horsemen of the Apocalypse. It will be important to spend more time preparing partners for forgiveness when there have been patterns of offenses. The couple's patterns will likely need to have some progress prior to beginning forgiveness work.

Relationship dynamics

Other relationship dynamics repair offenses are more troublesome: lack of emotional empathy, perceived lack of support, low self-esteem, general depressive mood, extreme distancer–pursuer patterns, explosive hair-trigger anger, and counter-anger. These factors can help therapists prognose how well partners will address their hurts positively. Motivation levels can vary widely. Some partners with considerable negative cognitive reactions to a partner's offenses may be ready to change habitual cognitive patterns in favor of repairing their relationship.

Let us suggest some questions to ask yourself as you address past hurts in relationships (see Intervention 19-2).

Intervention 19-2 Questions to Ponder as You Begin to Address Past Hurts with the Couple

1 What stage of change is each partner in? Baucom and his colleagues (Baucom et al., 2009) have proposed that partners move through three stages as they address offenses. They focused specifically on affairs, but their observations can be generalized to other offenses.

   1 First, partners tend to react to the offense. They seek to understand the *impact* of the offense. They essentially stop and try to intuit what has happened, what's been lost, and the threats that have arisen from the offense.
   2 Second, they seek to understand the *meaning* of the offense. Why did it happen? Could it have been prevented? If so, what could have prevented it? What will this mean to them individually? What will it mean to their relationship?
   3 Third, if their relationship survives the first two stages, they might work to *move on* from the offense. That can entail trying to repair the relationship, leave the relationship, or create a new standard for the relationship—three very different futures. Understanding where each partner is regarding the single big offense or the death-by-1000-paper-cuts is crucial to helping them move forward.

2 Is either partner moving to a quick but false repair? While grace, mercy, and forgiveness are valued, some partners quickly want to move past a huge relationship breach without considering justice, restitution, or even

the effect of the hurt on the relationship. This is similar to sustaining an athletic injury and rushing to resume the sport before healing has occurred. The chance of re-injury—or a worse injury—is high. After a major disruption in the relationship, partners need to take stock. The couple's therapist will likely facilitate that analysis.

3 How open are partners to trying to repair the damaged relationship? It would seem that's a no-brainer. It isn't. For some, the partner's affair has conceded the moral high ground. That high ground will be exploited by rubbing the partner's nose in it, threatening to divorce unless concessions are made, or punishing the person forever. If they agree to work on restoration, partners must talk about how much repair, apology, groveling, and restitution are necessary before the relationship might return to normal.

Stop rumination

Rumination is the attempt to gain a sense of understanding and control over an offense. The rumination may replay the event in their mind. Everything may remind the person of the offense, which makes the injustice gap *seem* larger than it is. It's like the brain is stuck in thinking about the offense. While it makes sense from a neurological perspective, why a brain might get stuck in a wicked problem like a major offense, it is also costly. Depression, binging behaviors, sleeping problems, substance abuse, and anxiety are all related to rumination. Eventually, friends get tired of hearing about the ruminating event, and it isolates people. Ev often calls it the "bad boy of mental health," and he is correct. Intervention 19-3 provides ways to help partners stop ruminating.

Intervention 19-3 Stopping Rumination

Help the person identify what is rewarding and costly about rumination. That can motivate change.

Education about rumination and its consequences can help move the offended person away from rumination.

Next, help partners engage in healthier thoughts, actions, and emotions. These can be distractions or thoughtful analyses of what good rumination does or doesn't do. If deeply stuck in rumination, some specific individual interventions may be needed from a trusted colleague or while the other partner supportively listens to the treatment activity. Medications can assist with ruminations if it is a broader problem beyond a specific event.

Some Actions to Reduce the Size of the Injustice Gap

We have developed many non-forgiveness ways partners could work independently (and together) to reduce the size of their injustice gaps. We highlight a few in this section thatyou can use help couples: tolerate the offense, forbear, offer restitution, give grace, practice radical acceptance, and use emotion to change the emotion.

Tolerate offensive behavior

One can decide to reduce the injustice gap by tolerating the partner's offensive behavior (see Intervention 19-4). That can reduce the partner's tendency to escalate hostilities. Toleration, however, is a double-edged sword. Because it simply squelches one's own responses, it can lead to frustration and a larger injustice gap. So, toleration is something we recommend only when partners seem to provoke each other whatever they do.

Intervention 19-4 Tolerate Offensive Behavior without Blowing Up

Ask partners for suggestions of ways they can self-soothe when they are upset. Discuss what works and what creates the least frustration.

Forbear responding negatively

Forbearance is toleration but (importantly) it is done *for the sake of the relationship, family, community, or other collective*. Having a positive reason for restraint sets forbearance apart from mere toleration. When partners forbear, they might choose to act kindly and patiently (see Intervention 19-5). In high-conflict couples, that might not be possible. So, merely not responding negatively might be all that the partner can manage. Collectivistic cultures often expect forbearance, emphasizing community needs above individual needs. Traditional religions also advocate forbearing as a spiritual response.

Intervention 19-5 Forbear Instead of Seeking Revenge (or Even Contemplating It)

First, get the partners to agree that forbearing can benefit the relationship. Emphasize that forbearance does not mean they will not work through conflicts. It means that partners choose to let some things slide for the good of the relationship.

Second, suggest that responding kindly and patiently are helpful but not necessary to forbearance, which is stifling negative responses for the good of the relationship. But ask whether there are ways partners can calm their anger and fear. For instance, many people recite the Serenity Prayer—"God, grant me the serenity to accept the things I cannot change, the courage to change the things I can, and the wisdom to know the difference"—to themselves is an emotion-regulation strategy, which is found in Psalms 29, 42, 91, and is also used in 12-step protocols.

From the field of psychotherapy, partners can work toward distress tolerance, radical acceptance, relaxation techniques, or loving-kindness cognitive interventions as ways to stay calm enough to forbear.

Offer or accept restitution

Restitution is seeking to make up for injustices, usually in kind. That is, if money was lost, restore money; if time was lost, do something to free up the other's time. Restitution helps people address the injustice gap in relationships. It is an antidote to revenge, which usually seeks to restore subjective feelings of justice by inflicting harm on the offender. Partners can offer restitution or request it politely. Making amends is perhaps a broader term than restitution, but they have a lot in common. Whereas restitution seeks to restore things to an equal status, making amends might not restore the previous status tit-for-tat. Instead, it might involve making up for what one has done to offend the other, often (but not always) through some incommensurable good, such as making up for money lost by working for the other person. A counselor can be useful in helping the couple determine a reasonable restitution plan (see Intervention 19-6) and perhaps remind partners of their plan if one partner tries to put it aside.

Intervention 19-6 Offer Restitution

What might restitution (or amends-making) look like? A partner might take on a chore for their partner, sell a personal item to cover a financial offense, buy a gift of something the offended has wanted, or earn extra income. To make amends, they might offer a public apology, create something valuable for the partner, or give time or resources to a charity the partner cares about.

Once a decision is made, barriers to implementing the plan need to be discussed. Some partners may begin to think negatively about the restitution, that their partner is "trying to buy their way out" of an offense. It's important to ensure that this isn't the only change necessary to rebuild trust and reconcile, but is intended to reduce the injustice gap. If the offender makes a heartfelt offer of restitution, and the offended rejects the offer, this may set the couple back. So good interventions are needed to help partners understand what accepting restitution means, discuss the meaning for both partners, be clear about their fears, and give the benefit of the doubt.

Give grace

People often say grace at mealtimes. But grace is broader. It is an act that can help reduce negative cycles of self-protection and defensiveness. Sells and Yarhouse (2011) define *grace* as an undeserved gift. Hodge et al. (2020) define *grace* as a gift of acceptance voluntarily given by an unobligated giver to an undeserving person.

Grace has been found to be associated with better mental health and interpersonal functioning (Hodge et al., 2020). We argue that grace applies well when there have been hurts in a relationship. While offering forgiveness can be an act of grace—an undeserved gift—there are many other ways people might treat offenses with kindness, generosity, or care. For example, when partners have argued throughout the day, one partner might make a special meal that night. It's natural to protect ourselves from harm. That is understandable. Acts of grace can short-circuit negative cycles and help couples begin to repair injustices (see Intervention 19-7).

Intervention 19-7 Grace Ain't Just for Supper

Credit for this intervention to Camden Morgante, PsyD, drawn from the relational grace theory of James Sells, Ph.D. (Sells & Yarhouse, 2011).

The first step is psychoeducation. Explain the concept of grace and ensure that the couple's problems fit with grace as an intervention. A worksheet with definitions of grace and the steps of this intervention can be found under worksheets on our website, www.hopecouples.com.

Second, locate inspirational narratives about grace.

- O. Henry's (1997) "The Gift of the Magi" is a good brief example.
- In the movie, *Les Misérables*, Jean Valjean steals some silver from a priest. He is caught. The priest not only tells the police that he hadn't stolen it, but he gives Valjean valuable silver candlesticks as an act of grace.
- Receiving grace demands a response. In *Captain Phillips* (2013), the mariner lead, played by Tom Hanks, is rescued and receives medical attention that saves his life. His gratitude is a dramatic response to grace. This movie is a reminder of the many small ways grace undergirds life through the care given by others.
- Therapists can search the web for further suggestions of movies you can direct the couple to watch, as part of their date night homework.

Step three is to discuss the grace practically enacted in their relationship. Here are some prompts.

- Has anyone in your life, now or historically, tended to give unmerited gifts? A family member, coach, teacher, neighbor, or friend perhaps?
- When have you shown grace to each other?
- Consider negative cycles or points of tension in your relationship. How might you extend grace to your partner when this tension comes up?
- What practical ways could you offer grace in an everyday way? What would it mean to you if your partner practiced grace to you?

Step four is homework. This brings application home to them. The goal is to have a positive experience of extending grace to break negative cycles. Good couple therapists can also help couples work through blocks and self-protective measures that extend negative cycles and prevent them from attempting acts of grace.

Practice radical acceptance

Some offenses, especially small to moderate ones, are unlikely to change. One partner may have ADHD, chronic depression, or difficult extended family dynamics. Sometimes, partners have to accept that the offense happened, look at it without avoidance, and admit that it will likely happen again. When partners learn that some offenses won't change, therapists can help promote radical acceptance (see Intervention 19-8 and Figure 19-1).

Intervention 19-8 Radical Acceptance

Therapists can coach couples in ways to come to terms with chronic issues. Practices such as relaxation, meditation/prayer, inspiring stories, scheduling acceptance, journaling, unified detachment of the problem, tolerance, or creating rule-governed strategies to communicate about the problem can help.

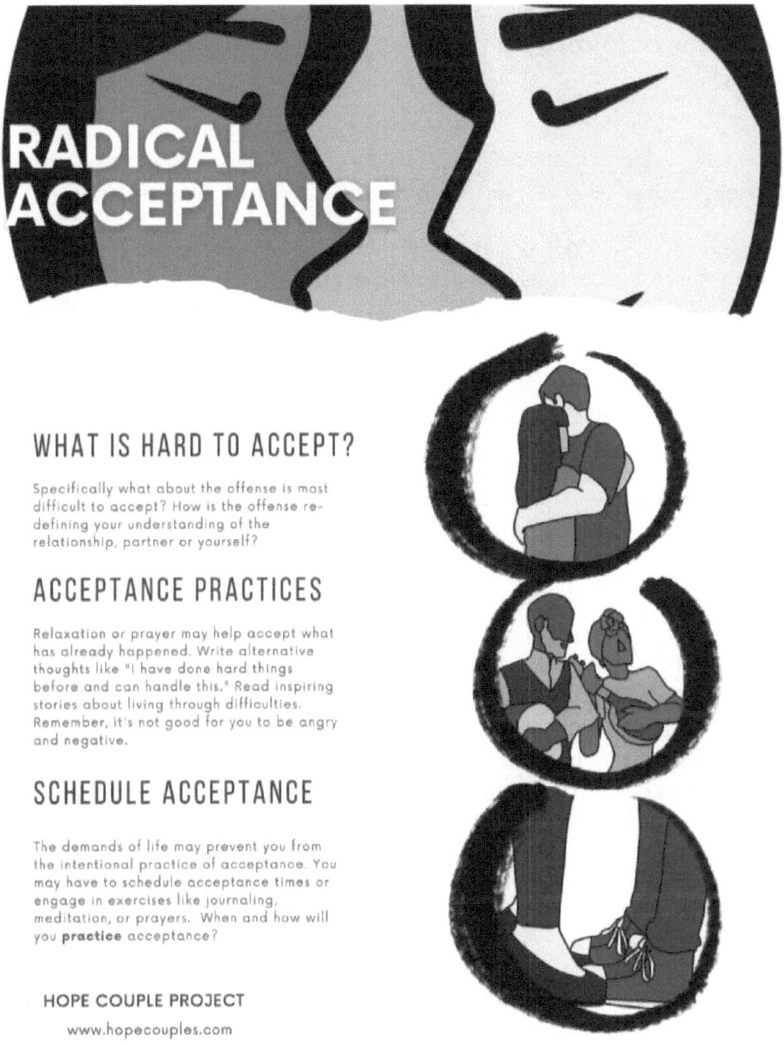
RADICAL ACCEPTANCE
WHAT IS HARD TO ACCEPT?
Specifically what about the offense is most difficult to accept? How is the offense re-defining your understanding of the relationship, partner or yourself?
ACCEPTANCE PRACTICES
Relaxation or prayer may help accept what has already happened. Write alternative thoughts like "I have done hard things before and can handle this." Read inspiring stories about living through difficulties. Remember, it's not good for you to be angry and negative.
SCHEDULE ACCEPTANCE
The demands of life may prevent you from the intentional practice of acceptance. You may have to schedule acceptance times or engage in exercises like journaling, meditation, or prayers. When and how will you **practice** acceptance?
HOPE COUPLE PROJECT
www.hopecouples.com

Figure 19-1 Radical Acceptance

Borrow a technique from emotion-focused therapy, transform emotion with emotion

When a partner is stuck in an emotional experience around offense or hurt, a couple's negative cycle can get extreme. The hurt and offense can get buried within the offended person and can be ensconced in the relationship dynamics. Emotion-focused couple therapy uses a technique called "transform emotion with emotion," which is compatible with various couple theories (see Intervention 19-9). Part of what is keeping the person stuck in one emotion is that they are blocking the unrecognized emotions. For instance, one partner shows anger to cover fear. The partner shows distress to cover anger. Uncovering the hidden emotion can be a breakthrough to intimacy.

Intervention 19-9 Transform Emotion with Emotion

To apply this, partners can ensure that when faced with a hot emotion situation, they can access *all* of the emotions and experiences, not just the felt emotions. In particular, frequent anger-only partners can find themselves lonely and isolated over time. If their goal is a long-term healthy relationship, accessing softer emotions like fear, sadness, compassion, and vulnerability can help build the bond between partners. The complex myriad of emotions is the more genuine and true experience of the event than the singular hard emotion.

Conclusion

In this chapter, we considered the injustice gap and some ways to reduce its size. We did not illustrate all of the ways to reduce the injustice gap. We only illustrated enough to give you a good idea of how you might do it. In the upcoming chapter, we move on to understanding forgiveness and how to use the REACH forgiveness intervention to promote forgiveness in individuals. In Chapter 21, we discuss how to use it directly with couples in session.

References

Baucom, D. H., Snyder, D. K., & Gordon, K. C. (2009). *Helping Couples Get Past the Affair: A Clinician's Guide*. New York: Guilford Press.

Fincham, F. D. Hall, J. & Beach, S. R. H. (2005). Forgiveness in marriage: Current status and future directions. *Family Relations, 55*, 415–427.

Henry, O. (1997). The Gift of the Magi. Simon & Schuster.
Hodge, A., Hook, J. N., Davis, D. E., Van Tongeren, D. R., Bufford, R. K., Bassett, R. L., & McMinn, M. R. (2020). Experiencing grace: A review of the empirical literature. *The Journal of Positive Psychology,* Advanced Online Publication. https://doi.org/10.1080/17439760.2020.1858943
Ripley, A. (2021). *High Conflict: Why We Get Trapped and How We Get Out.* Simon & Schuster.
Sells, J. N., & Yarhouse, M. A. (2011). *Counseling Couples in Conflict: A Relational Restoration Model.* IVP Academic.

20 Using an Effective Forgiveness Intervention

Teach Five Steps to REACH Forgiveness

Problem: Reducing the injustice gap needs forgiveness for most couples.
Solution: Use REACH model to support couple forgiveness.

On August 31, 1986, the Khian Sea (registered in Liberia), a sea-going cargo ship, was loaded with 14,000 tons of smoldering toxic ash from Philadelphia. The intent was to ship it to the Caribbean and dump it in the Bahamas. The Bahamas refused permission to dump. For 16 months, the Khian Sea searched for someplace in the Caribbean to unload its waste. It returned to Philadelphia. Pennsylvania refused to take back the waste.

In 1988, 4,000 tons were dumped in Haiti as "topsoil." When the Haitian government was informed, it ordered the ship to reload the waste, but the ship slipped away at night. It subsequently tried to unload the waste in Senegal, Morocco, Yugoslavia, Sri Lanka, and Singapore. In 1988, the ship was renamed the Pelicano (registered in Honduras) and secretly dumped its 10,000 remaining tons of toxic cargo in the Indian Ocean. Criminal charges were pressed, and eventually, the Pelicano was broken up.

After many attempts to get rid of the 4,000 tons of waste on its beaches, in November 1998, Haiti sent 2,500 tons to St. Lucie, FL, where it remained docked until 2000. Finally, Pennsylvania agreed to take back the by-now non-toxic waste and bury it in Franklin County, PA.

Troubled romantic relationships accumulate toxic waste over time. Both partners are like miniature Khian Seas, trying to offload as much toxicity as possible anywhere they can. The partner is the nearest dumping ground for each, but toxicity from a troubled marriage can be dumped to their children, extended families, workplaces, and community organizations.

DOI: 10.4324/9781003009382-24

Forgiveness can neutralize the toxicity of the waste that each partner has accumulated. When that happens, it gives partners a chance to reconcile. Reconciliation is a choice and has to be based on trustworthy accumulation of behaviors. But that's getting ahead of our story. We'll have to wait until Part 5 to get into reconciliation.

Understanding What Science Teaches about Forgiveness

In over 2,500 studies since the late 1990s, we've learned a lot about forgiveness. Before the late 1990s, forgiveness was usually considered religious because all five major religions valued it and encouraged their believers to practice it. But once the science of forgiveness exploded, people's understanding of forgiveness shifted. Now, it is typically embraced as a secular phenomenon. Secular refers to general acceptance by both religious and non-religious people. In this section, we describe what science knows about forgiveness and we organize it using a stress-and-coping theory of forgiveness (Worthington, 2006).

Hurts are accompanied by a sense of injustice—the injustice gap

Hurts are stressors, which people perceive as either challenges or threats. As described in Chapter 19, we keep an informal accounting of the degree of injustice-attending offenses. That accounting is part of our appraisal of the hurt. The injustice gap can be appraised as small or large, shrinking or growing, but its size is always directly related to the difficulty of dealing with the injustice. Unhappy partners are keenly aware of the pain from an injustice gap, whereas happier couples don't generally pay attention to it.

Hurts that are perceived as threats with large injustice gaps create stress reactions. These affect physiology, emotions, motivations, cognition, and behavioral intentions. Reactions can flare up and quickly be coped with. Or they can settle in. Unforgiveness is the overall name given to the suite of long-term stress reactions to a perceived injustice. We try to cope with stress by changing the stressor (i.e., what is causing the hurt), the appraisals (i.e., seeking to reduce, for example, the injustice gap), or the stress reactions (i.e., seeking to calm our physiology, lower emotions and negative motivations, change our cognition, and redirect our behavioral intentions).

There are many good ways to narrow the injustice gap as we saw in the previous chapter. Those are some of our coping mechanisms. People use their favorites, and that can reduce the size of the injustice gap to a size where forgiveness (another coping mechanism) might seem possible. An offender does not deserve forgiveness, so forgiveness is always an altruistic gift given by choice, not compulsion or coercion.

People use coping strategies to bring more justice into the relationship. Forgiveness is not opposed to justice. They act at different levels. Forgiveness is internal. Justice is social and societal. Thus, one can forgive internally and still pursue social or societal justice. Ev's mother was murdered on a cold New Year's Eve in 1996 (an internet search will find the full story told in videos). He found a path to forgive the young man who committed the murder. Yet, if the young man had ever been brought to justice, he would still be subject to the laws of the state prohibiting murder. Forgiveness is personal and internal. Justice is a social or societal system.

Scientists generally agree on their definitions of forgiveness. They see it as pro-social and benevolent responses to an offense or hurt. Beyond this general definition, there are smaller disagreements about what kinds of experiences hold priority when one forgives. Is it changes in effect, behavior, and cognition? Is it changes in motivations from avoidance and revenge motives to benevolent motives? Is it cognitive and behavioral changes? Is it changes in emotion and motivation? Is it changes in behavioral intentions? All of these change, and in many cases are bundled together. But scientists quibble about what are the most important changes. For therapy, it's better not to get embroiled in such controversies.

What forgiveness is not

While theorists might disagree about what forgiveness is, there is much agreement about what forgiveness is not. It is not forgetting. Forgiving requires remembering hurts, but remembering them differently. Forgiveness is not simply getting rid of unforgiveness by enacting justice, revenge, pay-back, or getting even. That means all of those alternatives to forgiveness we discussed in Chapter 19 are not forgiveness—not relinquishing the situation to God (for divine justice), not tolerating or forbearing, or accepting and moving on. Forgiveness is not psychologically manipulating one's understanding of the event by minimizing its importance, denying (i.e., psychologically refusing to admit to the truth of the offense), condoning (i.e., saying that the harm was acceptable), justifying (i.e., saying the offender acted rightfully), or excusing (i.e., saying that the offender had legitimate reasons for the offense). Forgiveness is also not reconciling, or restoring trust between two people, and is dependent on each trying sincerely to act trustworthily. It is not getting justice, which reduces the injustice gap.

Two Types of Forgiveness

We use two different types of forgiveness in our work with couples—emotional forgiveness and decisional forgiveness. *Emotional forgiveness* replaces negative, unforgiving emotions (resentment and bitterness) with positive, other-oriented emotions like empathy, sympathy, compassion, or love. Motivations are generally intertwined with emotions, so as replacement happens, motives change from avoidance or vengeance motives to more benevolent ones. *Decisional forgiveness* is a decision to put aside retaliation and treat the other person as more valued and valuable. So technically, decisional forgiveness is a behavioral intention statement that is valid regardless of whether the offender drops dead tonight and we never get to carry out the actual behavior. Emotional and decisional forgiveness are related to each other with a mean correlation coefficient of 0.4, which is not a high correlation and explains only 16 percent of the joint variation between them. So, they are not joined at the hip and while decisional forgiveness is often first for couples, it can occur in either order. Both emotional forgiveness and decisional forgiveness occur within people's skin.

In a nutshell, you now have the stress-and-coping theory of forgiveness. It is considered a "theory" because it has multiple models within it and a wealth of experimental evidence supporting it. It is the basis of a model for helping people who wish to forgive do so.

Using REACH Forgiveness

REACH (recall, empathy, altruistic gift, commit, and hold on) forgiveness is an intervention protocol—a scientific model that is more limited in scope than a theory because it aims just at how to help people forgive and does not attempt to explain the science of forgiveness.

It is evidence-based

It is supported by clinical science as an evidence-based treatment, whose uses are toward psychoeducational change for all types of unforgiveness and for people whose unforgiveness might be mild or very severe. It is not primarily a psychotherapeutic model, in that it is not targeted at psychopathology with unforgiveness at root. However, like many psychoeducational models, it is used frequently in individual psychotherapy and has some evidence supporting its effectiveness.

It is based on working through structured exercises to promote self-reflection

REACH forgiveness leads people through a set of experiences that will eventuate in their experiencing both emotional and decisional forgiveness. In addition, it seeks to help build a more forgiving personality (i.e., increase trait forgivingness).

It is delivered in a variety of ways

It is available as a psychoeducational group protocol. The other principal way REACH forgiveness is delivered is using individual DIY workbooks that take either 3.3 or 7 hours on the average.

It has been tested in conjoint couple therapy, and in sessions as part of a couple treatment plan. REACH forgiveness can be one potential part of reconciliation for couples needing to reconcile. Some partners are blocked by self-condemnation. REACH forgiveness using a DIY workbook can help a partner experience self-forgiveness.

REACH forgiveness is often adapted for individual psychotherapy and group psychotherapy, and a few studies have shown it effective in each. But its evidence-based support is exceptionally strong in psychoeducational groups (over 25 randomized controlled trials), DIY workbooks, couple therapy, and self-forgiveness DIY workbooks.

Use psychoeducational groups and DIY workbooks as adjuncts

Psychoeducational groups are good adjuncts to couple therapy. Or if a group isn't possible, partners can work through a DIY workbook to REACH forgiveness (available at no cost on **www.evworthington-forgiveness.com**). Working through the workbook independently of each other can forestall possible conflicts that might arise if they were in the same group together. We have found that just 10 minutes of session are needed to recommend the workbooks or groups and to deal with barriers to engaging with the workbook.

How to organize REACH forgiveness groups in a group practice

Organize groups and events to help clients, whether or not they are in couple therapy. There are many things you'll want to consider in creating a regular group program (see Intervention 20-1). Group programs for clients with interpersonal issues can be regularly run on one Saturday per month in a practice of four therapists.

Intervention 20-1 Issues to Consider as You Start a REACH Forgiveness Group Program for Your Practice

- We recommend that partners not attend forgiveness groups together if their target is forgiving offenses by each other. Most partners cannot manage the emotions that arise from being in the room with the partner. Often, only one partner needs the forgiveness group. That person can attend a group with others from the practice. Or both partners can use DIY workbooks.

- Screening issues: High-conflict partners can hijack the events if they haven't yet stabilized their relationship conflict.
- Goals: Informational talks can be done as a webinar or in person. Retreat weekends work well. Weekly groups for several weeks (not too many) need to solicit a written participation commitment.
- Process: It's nice to get couples to talk to each other after attending the group, but conflicts can occur if topics are power struggles.
- Evaluation: Try not to evaluate *only* satisfaction data. That tells you little about whether couples changed. Using goal-attainment scaling (GAS) can be helpful. GAS is a one-item scale at the end of treatment/program that asks whether people think they are acting better toward their partners: -2 is much less than anticipated; -1 somewhat less; 0 has reached reasonable expectations for improvement; +1 is somewhat exceeded; +2 has exceeded my expectations substantially.

Becoming qualified in using the REACH forgiveness protocol

Brace yourself. You don't need a boatload of continuing education or specialized training. You can use the REACH forgiveness protocol either formally in working through the protocol with a couple or informally by extracting the essence in working with the couple. Before launching into that, however, it would be vital to familiarize yourself with REACH forgiveness.

The easiest way to do this is to watch a two-hour video demonstration, which is for a six-hour group, boiled down to showing the group operation and discussing it in two hours. The demonstration is www.evworthington-forgiveness.com/run-groups. At the same time, you can follow along with the leader manuals, also available free on the website. You can select either the secular or Christian leader manual at the same web address. Participant manuals also are downloadable without cost.

Most interaction happens in the group between conversation partners. Facilitating the psychoeducational groups is not as complicated as group therapy. Pre-bachelors group leaders (supervised by a masters (MS) level clinical psychology practitioner) were almost as effective as post-MS practitioners. (There was a small though significant difference in effectiveness. There were no adverse reactions.)

What's in the REACH forgiveness protocol?

We provide a narrative summary of what is in the REACH forgiveness protocol in Intervention 20-2. We summarize point-by-point what is in the protocol. Still, if you plan to use this, we recommend visiting the website, perusing the free materials, and watching the training video.

Intervention 20-2 Point-by-Point Summary of the REACH Forgiveness Protocol

The "Five Steps" Preliminaries

- Identify one currently unforgiven transgression that you intend to work with throughout the intervention (called the target).
- Assess forgiveness using the forgiveness measures provided.
- Identify and narrate the hardest thing done to you that you successfully forgave.
- Reflect on an analogy of building a concrete, lasting structure.

Start the Intervention by Considering Forgiveness

- Reflect on the meaning of forgiveness through quotes.
- Commit to trying conscientiously to forgive.
- Define emotional and decisional forgiveness as two different types of forgiveness.
- There are benefits to forgiving, but paradoxically, you'll receive the most benefits if you try to forgive to give an *undeserved* gift of forgiveness to the target person.

How to Decisionally Forgive

- Invite decisional forgiveness. Few people are ready to do so at this point. We return to this after working through emotional forgiveness.

How to Emotionally Forgive

- Step R = Recall the Hurt (in Helpful Ways). Recall the hurt without excessive blame or dwelling on how you were victimized.
- Step E = Empathy for the One Who Hurt You. Emotionally replace negative emotions with positive ones. First, this reduces the negative (hopefully to zero). Then, you *may* go on to build a positive emotional valence. The positive replacement emotions *empathy, sympathy, compassion, altruistic love, or romantic love* all work.
- Step A = Altruism: Giving a Humble, Altruistic (Undeserved) Gift of Forgiveness. Get in touch with the gratitude we feel when we have been forgiven. Ask if they are ready to forgive the offender. Follow up with the more crucial question: What percent of the emotional unforgiveness am

I willing to release based on replacing it with better feelings (empathy, sympathy, compassion, or love) for the person?

- Step C = Commit to the Forgiveness you Experienced. Making this commitment memorable and public can help many partners. For example, they may write down their forgiveness, tell the therapist, or tell others.
- Step H = Hold on to Forgiveness (when you doubt). You'll experience reminders of the offense. Cover things the person can do to regulate negative emotions. Consider what to do when doubt occurs: Recall the analogy of being burned by a hot stove eye and getting near the heat: Pain does not equal unforgiveness. Distract yourself when rumination threatens.

How to Become a More Forgiving Person

- Complete twelve writing exercises to generalize learning to other unforgiven hurts or offenses.

Research Supporting REACH Forgiveness

Ev and Jen are trying not to burden this practice-oriented book with much research (see the bite-sized summary in Intervention 20-3). We hope this brief summary gives you confidence that this has a strong basis as an evidence-based treatment. The website www.evworthington-forgiveness.com has a list of forgiveness research that supports the REACH model.

Intervention 20-3 Research Supporting REACH Forgiveness Treatment

Almost 25 randomized controlled trials have been conducted worldwide on REACH forgiveness psychoeducational groups. Five studies have investigated the 7-hour DIY workbooks (4 secular, 1 Christian). One study, with 4,598 participants in China, Indonesia, Ukraine, Colombia, and South Africa, has investigated a 3.3-hour secular DIY workbook and found it effective (Ho et al., 2024). Most research on groups has been psychoeducational. However, two studies have dealt with people with psychological diagnoses seeking treatment (Sandage et al., 2015; Wade et al., 2018), and they compared Yalom-style process group therapy and the REACH forgiveness psychoeducational groups and found them equally effective.

REACH forgiveness has been incorporated in the hope-focused couple approach (HFCA) for treating couples, so it has been used in numerous tests of the HFCA. It has not been separated out from the whole treatment, except in Burchard et al. (2003), Ripley and Worthington (2002), and Worthington et al. (2015) for couple enrichment, and Ripley et al. (2014) and Ripley et al. (2021) for couple therapy, including a long-term (8 years) follow-up.

REACH forgiveness treatments consistently produce substantial forgiveness. But they also produce substantial increases in well-being, flourishing, and hope and decreases in depression and anxiety.

One large randomized controlled trial investigated a self-forgiveness DIY workbook (Griffin et al., 2015).

Conclusion

In this chapter, we described the REACH forgiveness intervention. But how is it used with couples? We discovered the hard way how not to use it. But we share how we can use it with couples in Chapter 21.

References

Burchard, G. A., Yarhouse, M. A., Kilian, M. K., Worthington, E. L., Jr., Berry, J. W., & Canter, D. E. (2003). A study of two marital enrichment programs and couples' quality of life. *Journal of Psychology & Theology, 31,* 240–252.

Griffin, B. J., Worthington, E. L., Jr., Lavelock, C. R., Greer, C. L., Lin, Y., Davis, D. E., & Hook, J. N. (2015). Efficacy of a self-forgiveness workbook: A randomized controlled trial with interpersonal offenders. *Journal of Counseling Psychology, 62*(2), 124–136.

Ho, M. Y., Worthington, E. L., Jr., Cowden, R. G., Bechara, A. O., Chen, Z. J., Gunatirin, E.Y., VanderWeele, T. J. (2024). International REACH forgiveness intervention: A multisite randomized controlled trial. *BMJ Public Health.* doi:10.1136/ bmjph-2023-000072

Ripley, J. S., Leon, C., Worthington, E. J., Berry, J. W., Davis, E. B., Smith, A., Atkinson, A., & Sierra, T. (2014). Efficacy of religion-accommodative strategic hope-focused theory applied to couples therapy. *Couple and Family Psychology: Research and Practice, 3,* 83–98.

Ripley, J., Solfelt, L., Ord, A., Garthe, R. C., Worthington, E. L., & Channing, T. (2021). Short- and long-term outcomes of hope-focused couple therapy. *Spirituality in Clinical Practice (Washington, D.C.).* https://doi.org/10.1037/scp0000286

Ripley, J. S., & Worthington, E. L., Jr. (2002). Hope-focused and forgiveness-based group interventions to promote marital enrichment. *Journal of Counseling and Development, 80,* 452–463.

Sandage, S. J., Long, B., Moen, R., Jankowski, P. J., Worthington, E. L., Jr., Rye, M. S., Wade, N. G. (2015). Forgiveness in the treatment of Borderline Personality

Disorder: A quasi-experimental pilot study. *Journal of Clinical Psychology*, *71*(7), 625–640.

Wade, N. G., Cornish, M. A., Tucker, J. R., Worthington, E. L., Jr., Sandage, S. J., & Rye, M. S. (2018). Promoting forgiveness: Characteristics of the treatment, the clients, and their interaction. *Journal of Counseling Psychology*, *65*(3), 358–371.

Worthington, E. L., Jr. (2006). *Forgiveness and Reconciliation: Theory and Application*. Brunner-Routledge.

Worthington, E. L., Jr., Berry, J. W., Hook, J. N., Davis, D. E., Scherer, M., Griffin, B. J., Wade, N. G., Yarhouse, M., Ripley, J. S., Miller, A. J., Sharp, C. B, Canter, D. E., & Campana, K. L. (2015). Forgiveness-reconciliation and communication-conflict-resolution interventions versus rested controls in early married couples. *Journal of Counseling Psychology*, *62*(1), 14–27.

21 Using REACH Forgiveness in Session

Walk Couples Through It

Problem:	Couples want to forgive each other, but feel stuck in moving toward forgiveness, especially emotional forgiveness.
Solution:	Use faith, work, and valuing love to promote a journey of forgiveness.

Forgiveness with couples is hard work. Both are usually offenders and offended. Severity of offenses can be uneven. One partner may be ready to forgive and move forward, while the other is insecure about forgiveness. They easily get caught in the blame game, defending themselves and further damaging the relationship.

Many therapists avoid forgiveness work with couples because of these dynamics. Yet leaving major hurts or patterns of hurts unaddressed is like leaving an infection in hopes that it will heal. It might. Or not. With couples, unforgiveness might travel through the duo and undo all the good work of stabilization, hopeful interaction, and bonding. We can't omit forgiveness from the treatment plan.

Treating Unforgiveness Using REACH Forgiveness

We have recommended REACH forgiveness for your use. It is the most researched psychoeducational group and do-it-yourself (DIY) workbook treatment available, and it has been investigated and shown to be effective with couple enrichment and therapy.

It's not the most investigated treatment for individual psychotherapy. Although it is aimed at forgiving troublesome events—with far and away the preponderance of evidence supporting it—studies of it have

DOI: 10.4324/9781003009382-25

not often targeted psychopathology. Exceptions have been published, showing success with people diagnosed with borderline personality disorder (Sandage et al., 2015) and community adults seeking outpatient group psychotherapy (Wade et al., 2018). So, there is some evidence that REACH forgiveness can work in more focused psychotherapy for hurts and offenses.

Forgiveness therapy targeted at very serious individual problems

The research base for REACH forgiveness is not targeted at serious, traumatic, or highly disturbed clients. Problems like incest are likely better matched with long-term individual forgiveness therapy (Enright & Fitzgibbons, 2015). Serious psychopathology, like PTSD or personality disorder, requires full individual assessment to ensure each partner is stable enough to withstand couple therapy and forgiveness work. Even in regular couple therapy, we put off dealing with forgiveness until the relationship has improved. In our clinic, we usually start the forgiveness stage after about six to ten sessions of general couple therapy.

Couple therapy for infidelity

Similarly, some couple issues require more targeted treatments. Infidelity is one of those. The wise practitioner does not simply rely on their experience but supplements it with people who have made this a specialty. The team of Kristina Coop Gordon, Donald H. Baucom, and Douglas K. Snyder developed a specialty treatment for infidelity. They have created resources for both the therapist (Baucom et al., 2009) and the couple themselves (Snyder et al., 2023).

Walking through REACH forgiveness in a conjoint couple session

Before beginning to work with couples on forgiveness, there are some things for you to know. The most important is that both partners have been both offenders and victims. That does not mean that the big recent infidelity (for example) can be blown off because the other person has forgotten to take out the trash in the past. Those big events must be dealt with! The other important starting point is that not every offense must be explicitly apologized for and forgiven.

In any relationship of any length—not just troubled ones—there are all too many accumulated hurts and offenses. Each person has inflicted the hurts. So, each partner is a victim of many offenses and an offender who has inflicted many offenses and hurts.

We know that sounds daunting. But the good news is that partners do not have to deal with every hurt to feel that they have forgiven the partner. When people say they can't forgive *their partner*, they usually mean that they have experienced many hurts and offenses—so many that it no longer makes sense to name each one. Generalization has occurred from individual hurts to the partner as the offender.

Forgiveness takes advantage of this same generalization. That is, what will likely be important is for partners to (eventually) identify the three or so most significant hurts or offenses. Those will signify or symbolize all of the lesser offenses. If the big three (usually) can be forgiven, for most people, generalization will occur, and the person might conclude that they forgive *the partner*.

Because partners want to reduce the size of the injustice gap, they will likely want to apologize for the hurts they inflicted and make restitution or amends for their offense. Just like the offenses can generalize, forgiveness can also generalize across patterns of offenses. So, not every offense or hurt needs to be explicitly apologized for and repaired through amends. That should not be taken as a "rule." If a partner needs an apology for a particular hurt, it should be given freely, regardless of whether this is the first hurt dealt with or the fifty-first.

Step-by-step through teaching partners REACH forgiveness

REACH forgiveness is effective with early married community-based couples (Worthington et al., 2015). The REACH forgiveness part of the hope-focused couple approach (HFCA) has also been supported, as we presented in the previous chapter. As you plan to use REACH forgiveness (see Figure 21-1), consider an intensive model for some couples, with a double or even triple session to spend time on forgiveness. This will help the couple move through REACH in one sitting, which we think is beneficial to the couple's progress. If this isn't an option in your practice, break up the work across 2-3 sessions. Cramming in the emotional learning won't benefit the couple.

Choose four target transgressions to work with (see Intervention 21-1)

Each partner chooses four hurts. That provides enough grist for the mill to both learn and apply the method. One of the four will be from the past before they formed their relationship. Three will be from their relationship. REACH forgiveness is learned on a specific offense or hurt rather than learned as a general abstract program. Thus, partners must identify hurts so that they can learn how to forgive using this evidence-based method.

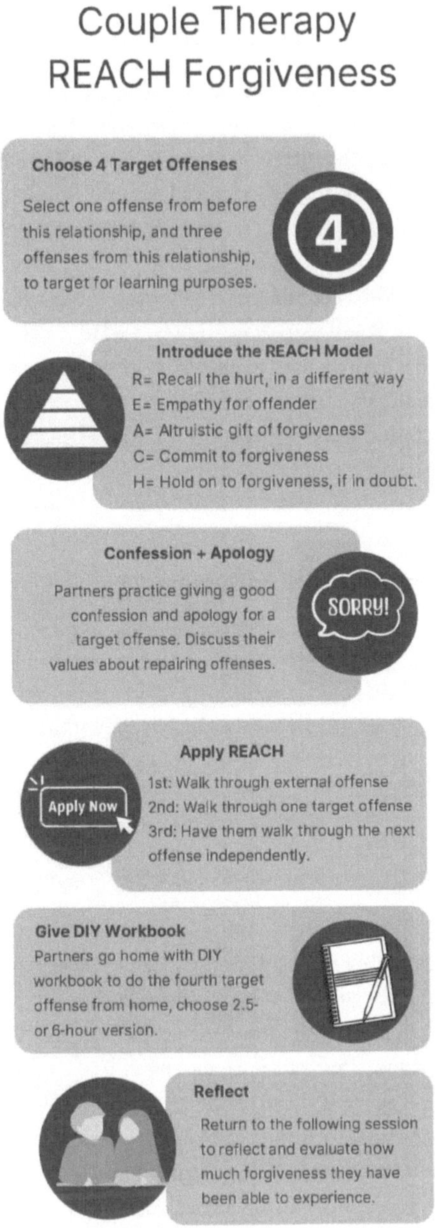

Figure 21-1 Four Interventions 21-1, 21-2, 21-3, and 21-4 to Promote Movement toward Reconciliation

Intervention 21-1 Choose Four Offenses to Work On

To do the full intervention, the couple will need all four offenses, one from the past, outside their relationship, and three from their relationship.

Each partner has veto power over offenses. Remind them that the offense can't be so overwhelming that they can't learn the model. If either partner feels like it's overwhelming, they can veto it. Let them pick one partner to start.

When partners have accumulated significant hurts and offenses over a long period together, you'll usually go slowly. Spend more time teaching the REACH forgiveness method on events before the partners met. Even if they have a long-term history, use events before they became romantically involved. This way, one person can be the (first) designated learner, and the other can be supportive.

Introduce REACH forgiveness (see Intervention 21-2)

While most people are familiar with forgiveness—perhaps through movies, books, or religious experiences—they are not necessarily familiar with the REACH forgiveness model. So, teaching is in order. In a conjoint session, you'll teach one partner while the other is designated helper. Then, the helper will try it.

Intervention 21-2 Introduce the REACH Forgiveness Model

Once the pre-relationship transgression is chosen by each partner, make the roles clear. You might begin, "I'll talk you through this, but you (Susan) will be applying this. You (Rodney) will be practicing empathy and support."

Do some initial education with both partners. If you haven't already talked about the injustice gap, you might want to frame the work with that concept. Begin with the essential information that holding onto unforgiveness has been shown to cause rumination, which is bad for mental health, poisons relationships, such as child or workplace relationships, even if the unforgiven hurts are with a partner, and even has physical health effects like higher blood pressure and stress. Forgiving yields benefits of removing the ill effects of unforgiveness and also provides positive effects beyond that. It broadens perspectives, builds resources, promotes flourishing, and provides forgivers with a sense of well-being. People who forgive are better off in many ways than people who hold grudges or seek vengeance. If you cover the information in this paragraph, you'll already help partners begin to forgive.

There are two *separate* types of forgiveness. The REACH forgiveness method is just a structured way of helping people experience each. Explain that decisions to forgive govern intentions not to pay the other person back, but to treat the person more humanly and humanely. Suggest that people can commit to such intentions and carry them out, yet still feel emotionally upset when recalling the hurt. Ask whether that has ever happened to them.

Say that this suggests that there are two different types of forgiveness. The other type is emotional forgiveness, which replaces negative resentments toward the person who hurt you with positive emotions like empathy, sympathy, compassion, or love.

Tell them that it doesn't matter what order the decision or emotional peace occur in. Often, people make a decision and that leads to more emotional peace. But if people do things to replace unforgiveness with more positive emotions, it makes decisions easier to carry out. The REACH forgiveness model will walk you through the emotional forgiveness and then ask whether, now that you feel differently toward the person, you might want to decide that you'll treat them differently.

So, what is the REACH model? A graphic can be helpful here. REACH stands for: Recall the hurt; Empathy; Altruistic gift of forgiveness; Commit to forgiveness you experience; and Hold onto forgiveness when you doubt. This is a good point to address misunderstandings or resistance to forgiveness concepts, so it's important not to rush through the education step.

Set up the move to reconciliation that you'll cover in detail in later sessions

Forgiveness happens inside us, but reconciliation happens in the way we treat each other—and that can affect whether we forgive. So, before applying forgiveness, tell the partners that you want to touch on part of reconciliation—confessing and offering apologies—because that is sometimes what the offender does, before we even consider forgiving. These two activities are so central to intimate partner forgiveness that it would be unwise to skip them.

In Intervention 21-3, we discuss the importance of giving and receiving a good apology (or, more generically, a good confession). Generally, partners will have an easier time dealing with an offense if the partner has made a good confession (including an apology). A good confession contains a good apology plus empathy, an offer of amends, and a request for forgiveness. As we know, a good confession will narrow the injustice gap, making forgiving easier. Emphasize that you will spend more time on confessions and apologies later, as you talk more about reconciliation.

Intervention 21-3 Practice Confession and Apology

The partners can select one offense to confess and apologize for. Before both partners apply the REACH forgiveness model, we want to touch on what a good confession and good apology are.

You'll need to use your clinical judgment here. You can suggest to partners that they can confess and apologize for some actual hurts they inflicted on each other (if you think that the partners have largely conquered power struggles). If they have residual power struggles in which they have an underlying issue about who has the power, you might not want to have them try to practice on an actual hurt in their relationship. Instead, choose a hypothetical wrong—like a forgotten task or careless remark. Get each partner to give what they consider to be a good apology. It should be sincere, remorseful, specific, and sensitive to the pain that the behavior caused.

At this point, couples often need to clarify intent versus impact. For example, a forgotten birthday might have happened because the partner who forgot was overwhelmed with stress from multiple events. The intent was good (and the partner might have purchased a birthday present a week ago), but the circumstances overwhelmed the intent. On the other hand, the forgetful partner must also recognize that the impact on the partner might be way out of line with the forgetful partner's experience. For the forgotten partner, this might signify a slide into neglect that she grew up with. Both partners need to consider both the intent and impact of the event. The pain can be real, even if it was not intentionally inflicted.

You might teach about good confessions, which is optional, depending on time and whether the apology was relatively good. If the apology is not helpful, the you might want to teach about what good confessions entail. This is covered in Part 5 on reconciliation.

Apply the REACH method several different ways (Intervention 21-4)

First, each tries to forgive the pre-relationship hurt while being encouraged by the partner. Second, manage overly optimistic expectations. Third, have them review their learning by teaching you the concepts. Fourth, tackle one current hurt in their own relationship. Fifth, instead of using the structure, use the ideas on the second current hurt (which is the third of four hurts to which they are applying the method).

Intervention 21-4 Apply REACH

Forgive the pre-relationship hurt. Have the person working (Susan in our example) try to work through some brief exercises to forgive the person who hurt her prior to ever meeting Rodney. Coach Rodney to encourage successes. You might try an empty-chair exercise to help Susan empathize with her offender. Ask whether she understands the offender better, and if so, does she feel differently toward the offender. Observe that she R (recalled the hurt) when she thought up the offense to work on, and the empty-chair helped her begin to E (empathize). Then, considering her feelings now, she considered whether to give an A (altruistic gift of forgiveness).

Manage expectations. Point out that the amount of forgiveness experienced clearly is proportional to the amount of time spent focused on forgiving. She spent little time and so probably it would be surprising if much emotional forgiveness was experienced. Once some forgiveness is experienced, invite the learner to decide to treat the person differently or, if the person is no longer available, to decide that they would treat the person differently if the person were here. The point here is to learn the method, not experience life-altering forgiveness. Let Rodney go through the same experiences with his pre-relationship offense.

Have them teach the concepts. Ask the partners to teach you three things before moving forward to their offenses. The first is, what is emotional forgiveness; the second is, what is decisional forgiveness; the third is, what are the REACH steps?

Apply the method to an existing hurt of each. "We now come to the hard part. We want to apply this to some hurts you still hold and don't believe are fully emotionally forgiven. You have each selected three hurts that still rankle, and you still get negative emotions when you think about them. So, we'd like to have you practice on a couple of those. How does that sound?"

"The idea here is that you don't have to forgive all 1000 small offenses since you met to forgive each other thoroughly. If you each choose three offenses that bother you and apply this method to those, you might feel that forgiving those is 'good enough' to consider that you have forgiven your partner. How does that sound?"

Then, the other person chooses one and works through REACH, forgiving that offense. They work through the hurt from their perspectives first and then from the other.

Discuss the third offense. Have the couple have a free-wheeling discussion of the third offense, first by one partner and then by the other. If there is enough time remaining in the session, partners can try these actions taught and practiced in a structured sequence under the watchful eye of the therapist. The acid test is whether they can apply the principles without structure. So, one partner, then the other, initiates discussing their one remaining offense. After the first partner tries to forgive, with (hopefully) a good confession by the offender to start the ball rolling, the therapist can get the partners to review their performance. After that debriefing, the other partner tries to forgive their third offense, and another debriefing occurs.

Have both partners work through a DIY workbook (Intervention 21-5)

The six-hour psychoeducational group format was adapted to a DIY workbook that took 6 to 7 hours to complete. The reason was to increase portability so that forgiveness psychoeducation could scale up to public and mental health. It was adapted as an internet intervention in Australia (Nation et al., 2018). Recently, a large randomized controlled trial (RCT) involving 4,598 participants from Hong Kong, Indonesia, Ukraine (two sites), Colombia, and South Africa found the REACH forgiveness 2- to 3-hour DIY workbooks effective (Ho et al., 2024).

The brief DIY REACH forgiveness workbooks are available without cost in English, Spanish, Chinese (Standard), Ukrainian, and Indonesian (see https://reach.discoverforgiveness.org). Workbooks and Ev's personal webpage are available at www.evworthington-forgiveness.com.

Intervention 21-5 Work through a Do-It-Yourself Workbook on REACH Forgiveness

It is helpful for partners to work independently through a DIY workbook on REACH forgiveness. Several free workbooks are available—a 3-hour secular version, a 6- to 7-hour secular version, and a 7-hour Christian version. Use your clinical discernment to decide which to recommend. A major clinical question is the timing of doing the workbook. Some therapists prefer to assign the workbook the week before the forgiveness session. That can save time because the partners (if they have completed the workbook) will have already thought through the model, and the teaching done during the session will be reviewed. However, other couple therapists like to use it to reinforce the learning during the session. They assign the workbook after the first forgiveness session. That way, the session seems fresh, and learning is interpersonal, and any misconceptions can be immediately corrected. We have done it both ways. Both have benefits. And costs.

Have partners reflect on their learning

The "Hold onto Forgiveness" portion is especially important for couples who have worked on forgiveness. Ask them to review that portion of the DIY manual or participant manual (if in a group). Process learning within the session (see Intervention 21-6). Predict that they will experience some unforgiveness in the weeks following the intervention, especially when feeling tension in the relationship or stress.

Intervention 21-6 Have Partners Reflect on Their Learning

Get the partners to process their experience. Due to time constraints, you might do this in the session following completion of the DIY workbook.

Ask prompting questions. What part did they find most difficult? Where did they get relief in forgiveness? Did they feel relief in being forgiven?

If plagued with self-forgiveness struggles, then adding a self-forgiveness module can be helpful. Don't rush through processing. This reflection solidifies experiential learning from the in-session and DIY workbooks.

Use Socratic questioning to help illuminate issues that still need resolution.

Wrong-Doing and Wrong-Being with Offenders

Besides forgiving the partner, each partner might need self-forgiveness for their offenses. Recent research on forgiveness has moved beyond merely understanding the processes a person goes through when trying to forgive a wrong done to them. Instead, researchers and clinicians have seen that forgiveness happens in a context that involves how the offender and victim talk about transgressions. This will be covered in depth in our discussion of forgiveness and reconciliation through experiencing empathy (FREE) in Part 5, so we will not cover it here. Instead, we will look at a relatively common offender experience—self-condemnation.

Many methods of confronting one's wrong-doing

The most recent *Handbook of Forgiveness, 2nd edition* (Worthington & Wade, 2020) revealed a clear trend. About one-third of the chapters' authors called for more attention to the offender. Many mentioned guilt-management methods, reconciliation, making amends, apologizing, or asking for forgiveness. Several mentioned ways offenders deal with their offenses psychologically, such as accepting one's imperfections, self-compassion, and self-forgiveness. Others mentioned equanimity-producing methods like mindfulness to deal with shame.

Dealing with shame and guilt of wrong-being when offenders believe they have not committed a moral wrong

Self-condemnation and perhaps accompanying guilt and shame might still be experienced, even though a person feels they have done no moral wrong. For example, a person might feel guilt, shame, and self-condemnation because the relationship is flailing, believing they did not do enough to save it—taking all of the responsibility for the relationship's outcome on the self. Or the person might feel self-condemnation because their mental health disorder stresses the relationship.

Promoting self-forgiveness in individuals

Virtually all of the writing on self-forgiveness has been aimed at individuals working through self-forgiveness using either a DIY workbook, individual psychotherapy, or group therapy. In interventions by Cornish and Wade (2015) in individual psychotherapy or Griffin et al. (2015) using DIY workbooks, treatments are based on self-condemnation usually because others have been injured or offended. Consideration of the effects on others is part of the overall therapeutic protocol. But in this section, we will summarize the Griffin et al. (2015) intervention (see Intervention 21-7), which can be used in psychotherapy, conjoint couple therapy, group therapy, or as a DIY workbook. The idea is that, if wrongs have been done, the wrongdoer must deal responsibly with spiritual disruption (Step 1) due to the wrong-doing and also with damage done to both others (Step 2) and psychologically to oneself (such as moral injury; Step 3). Then, the person can work through the emotional self-forgiveness and make a decision to forgive the self (Step 4). Self-acceptance (Step 5) often needs special attention because one can forgive oneself for hurtful actions but might still struggle to accept oneself as a person capable of such hurtful acts. In Step 6, the person commits to not repeating the hurtful behavior.

Intervention 21-7 Six Steps to Decisional plus Emotional Self-Forgiveness

You can teach this quickly in therapy.

Responsibility

Step 1: Receive God's Forgiveness (or Humanity, or Nature)—Moral repair (Decisional)
Step 2: Repair Relationships—Moral repair (Decisional)
Step 3: Reduce Rumination (Rumination, Expectations, Standards)—Internal condemnation (Emotional)

Forgive Yourself

Step 4: Explicit Decision plus REACH Emotional Self-forgiveness—Moral Repair (Decisional) plus Internal condemnation (Emotional)

Repair of Self

Step 5: Realize Self-Acceptance—Internal condemnation (Emotional)
Step 6: Resolve to Live Virtuously—Moral Repair (Decisional)

Dealing with self-condemnation when no moral wrong has been committed

Jemimah Rohini Bem and Peter Strelan at the University of Adelaide (Australia) have been working on an intervention to promote self-forgiveness using an adapted Six Steps to REACH Self-Forgiveness protocol to forgive non-moral offenses. The project will be Bem's dissertation. She analyzed the differences between treating moral and non-moral self-condemnation and concluded that the six steps that included REACH forgiveness could still form a viable treatment; however, some changes had to be made (see Intervention 21-8).

Intervention 21-8 An Intervention to Forgive Oneself Due to Non-Moral Self-Condemnation

Even though Bem and Strelan found that the same steps were needed to handle self-condemnation with or without doing something morally wrong, they concluded that some of the steps needed reordering. For example, Bem has people deal with the Sacred (Step 1) and their psychological issues (Step 3). The step of making social repairs is skipped initially because other people have not necessarily been negatively affected by non-moral self-condemnation. Step 4 (Emotional self-forgiveness and decisional forgiveness) is done next. Self-acceptance (Step 5) is still a problem, as is committing not to fall back into the trap of self-condemnation again. But now, at last, comes the analysis of whether one's own self-absorption has made social demands on others, and Step 2 is now the last step in the protocol.

Working with one partner on self-forgiveness in conjoint therapy

The intrapsychic dynamics of why a person might experience excessive self-condemnation within a couple's relationship can be complex. If a therapist is not oriented toward psychodynamic therapy, the therapist might not want to delve into those motives in couple therapy. Even seeing self-condemnation as a functional impairment to the relationship might be something most therapists want to avoid, if they are committed to couple dynamics instead of individual dynamics. But sometimes, we are forced to deal with self-forgiveness because self-condemnation is interfering with couple therapy. For example, excessive self-blame might functionally induce a person to facilitate irresponsibility in the partner because the self-punitiveness of self-blame might forestall needed criticism of the partner.

But, suppose we have a personality-driven self-condemnation that is not localized to the dynamics of the relationship but pervades multiple relationships. The partners believe that they need to deal with it in couple therapy. Let's say the partners agree (and it fits with your clinical judgment) that one partner is self-condemning, which is affecting the relationship. In Intervention 21-9, we consider working with one of the partners.

Intervention 21-9 Working with One Partner on Curbing Their Excessive Self-Condemnation

Let's say the partners agree (and it fits with your clinical judgment) that one partner is self-condemning which is affecting the relationship. You might want to focus on that patient, with the partner being treated as a support to assist the patient's progress. You can help the patient work through the six steps, with the supportive partner being coached to provide support but not to take on the role of a "junior clinician." We might exert as much effort toward showing the supportive partner what to do and not to do, as teaching the other partner how to apply the six steps to their problems.

Conclusion

Many forgiveness resources have been developed so individuals could examine themselves and forgive more quickly and thoroughly than if they relied on non-evidence-based methods. In the present chapter, we have described how to help partners in conjoint couple therapy forgive. This involves carefully working with them as a couple. But forgiveness takes time. And much of that time must simply be spent alone, as an individual in a group, so partners' involvement with forgiving requires effort outside of therapy sessions.

Forgiving is about repairing damaged emotional bonds, which is essential for ensuring a strong emotional bond exists. In the next part of the book, we look to rebuild the emotional bond through reconciliation.

References

Baucom, D. H., Snyder, D. K., & Gordon, K. C. (2009). *Helping Couples get Past the Affair: A Clinician's Guide*. New York: Guilford Press.

Cornish, M. A., & Wade, N. G. (2015). A therapeutic model of self-forgiveness with intervention strategies for counselors. *Journal of Counseling & Development, 93*, 96–104. doi:10.1002/j.1556-6676.2015.00185.x.

Enright, R. D., & Fitzgibbons, R. P. (2015). *Forgiveness Therapy: An Empirical Guide for Resolving Anger and Restoring Hope*. Washington, DC: American Psychological Association.

Griffin, B. J., Worthington, E. L., Jr., Lavelock, C. R., Greer, C. L., Lin, Y., Davis, D. E., & Hook, J. N. (2015). Efficacy of a self-forgiveness workbook: A randomized controlled trial with interpersonal offenders. *Journal of Counseling Psychology, 62*(2), 124–136.

Ho, M. Y., Worthington, E. L., Jr., Cowden, R. G., Bechara, A. O., Chen, Z. J., Gunatirin, E. Y. . . . & VanderWeele, T. J. (2024). International REACH forgiveness intervention: A multisite randomized controlled trial. *BMJ Public Health*. doi:10.1136/ bmjph-2023-000072

Nation, J. A., Wertheim, E. H., & Worthington, E. L., Jr (2018). Evaluation of an online self-help version of the REACH forgiveness program: Outcomes and predictors of persistence in a community sample. *Journal of Clinical Psychology, 74*(6), 819–838. https://doi.org/10.1002/jclp.22557

Sandage, S. J., Long, B., Moen, R., Jankowski, P. J., Worthington, E. L., Jr., Rye, M. S., Wade, N. G. (2015). Forgiveness in the treatment of Borderline Personality Disorder: A quasi-experimental pilot study. *Journal of Clinical Psychology, 71*(7), 625–640.

Snyder, D. K., Gordon, K. C. & Baucom, D. H. (2023). *Getting Past the Affair: A Program to Help you Cope, Heal, and Move On—Together or Apart. (2nd edition)* Guilford Press.

Wade, N. G., Cornish, M. A., Tucker, J. R., Worthington, E. L., Jr., Sandage, S. J., & Rye, M. S. (2018). Promoting forgiveness: Characteristics of the treatment, the clients, and their interaction. *Journal of Counseling Psychology*, *65*(3), 358–371.

Worthington, E. L., Jr., Berry, J. W., Hook, J. N., Davis, D. E., Scherer, M., Griffin, B. J., Wade, N. G., Yarhouse, M., Ripley, J. S., Miller, A. J., Sharp, C. B, Canter, D. E., & Campana, K. L. (2015). Forgiveness-reconciliation and communication-conflict-resolution interventions versus rested controls in early married couples. *Journal of Counseling Psychology*, *62*(1), 14–27.

Worthington, E. L., Jr., & Wade, N. G. (Eds.). (2020). *Handbook of Forgiveness, 2nd ed*. Routledge.

Part 5

Reconciling and Rebuilding

22 Teaching Forgiveness and Reconciliation

Guide Partners through Four Steps to Set Partners FREE

Problem:	Once repairs have occurred, there is still a need to intentionally reconcile in a relationship.
Solution:	Use FREE interventions to help couples forgive and reconcile.

Dani and David had done good work moving past old hurts. They had listened and shown some empathy. Empathy was hard for them, especially for Dani, who had a pile-up of childhood hurts from her parents. They were still wary of each other and feared they would fall back into old patterns. They had established a new dynamic by working hard in therapy.

But they didn't feel reconciled. They walked on eggshells every time there was anger or disconnection in the relationship. They had decided to be forgiving toward each other, but fear lurked in the cupboards and corners of their relationship.

We set the stage at the beginning of Part 5 by describing the Bridge to Reconciliation, which is the core of the intervention called FREE—forgiveness and reconciliation through experiencing empathy. FREE is a four-step procedure involving deciding that the partners want to reconcile, discussing the transgression, detoxing the relationship if it had begun to deteriorate, and putting devotion back into the relationship. In this chapter, we provide an overview of FREE. We break down the steps in the other three chapters in Part 5.

DOI: 10.4324/9781003009382-27

The FREE Intervention

The FREE intervention is a complex intervention that helps couples both forgive and reconcile (see Figure 22-1). Reconciliation occurs in four steps:

1. Decision: Should we reconcile, and if so, when and how?
2. Discussion: How do people ask their partner to explain something that seems to have been wrong-doing, and how do people make a good confession?
3. Detoxification: How do we remove the poison from estrangement, which might be years in duration? and
4. Devotion: How do we devote ourselves to positive love?

Ev has laid these out in *Forgiveness and Reconciliation: Theory and Application* (Worthington, 2006), which fits the interventions within a stress-and-coping theory of forgiveness (see Chapter 20). The REACH forgiveness intervention is thoroughly integrated within the stress-and-coping model of forgiveness. Chapter 20 provides a complete description of REACH forgiveness and Chapter 21 shows how to work with couples to use it in couple therapy.

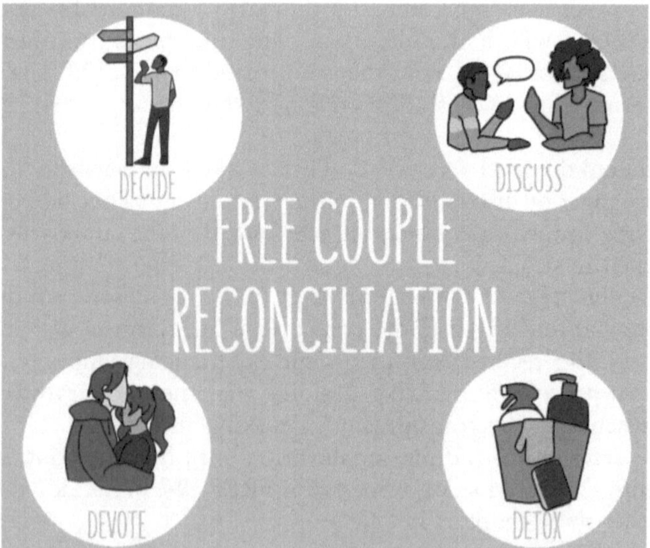

Figure 22-1 Four Steps to Forgiveness and Reconciliation through Experiencing Empathy (FREE)

Where FREE fits with treating couples

By the time the couple has progressed through couple therapy to deal with forgiveness and reconciliation, they should be stabilized and growing. The initial phase of therapy requires solidifying the working relationship between the therapist and the couple, assessing the problems, and collaborating on a treatment plan. Generally, before engaging the FREE intervention partners are feeling fairly good about the therapy relationship and the prospects for therapy. They are regaining hope for their relationship in general and for the prospect of therapy being effective. Paradoxically, some couples can feel so good here that they seek to terminate. If they do, their gains will often be short-lived, and they will conclude that therapy did not work. As we cautioned earlier, such premature termination can usually be avoided by alerting the partners ahead of time that this is a motivational shift whose best function is to energize them to tackle the hard work during the second phase of therapy. There, they deal with conflict resolution, communication, and intimacy.

At the end of the second phase of therapy, they will likely see symptomatic relief. Again, the tendency is to feel good enough to skip the third phase of therapy, in which they have to deal with difficult past behaviors and work through forgiveness, reconciliation, and termination. Again, anticipating this potential dropout point, the therapist can alert people to the temptation to drop out prematurely. That warning should come during the feedback session early in therapy but should be repeated as therapy moves to its end game.

The third phase of treatment is aimed at FREE, followed by termination rituals and a final assessment and feedback. The third phase of therapy is not like phase two, which tends to feature problem-solving that changes patterns of conflict, communication, and intimacy. The FREE phase of couple therapy deepens work done earlier, making it more specific to dealing with past hurts and making sure reconciliation is thorough. It aims at fostering lasting functionality and therefore repeats—but differently—some of the things that were practiced during phase two. It is structured around the four tasks of FREE: decisions about reconciliation, discussions of transgressions, detoxifying the relationship of poisonous past emotions around previous offenses, and developing a renewed dedicated devotion to the relationship.

Decide to Reconcile (Step 1)

In this step, we describe decisions that couples must make regarding when, where, and how to try to reconcile. We help the therapist know how to promote productive decisions.

Decisions about reconciling

Preparations to try to reconcile are important. Jen designed this educational intervention to help couples *prepare* to forgive and reconcile by discussing their previous experiences with forgiveness and reconciliation. Some people have negative experiences with forgiveness, which can set up a failure if these experiences are unexplored. The therapist can convey the basic principles of forgiveness through three memorable ideas (see Interventions 22-1, 22-2, and 22-3). These deal with war, a Star Wars metaphor, and whiskey. We emphasize couple-led discussion more in this phase than in previous phases. However, couples might use a written worksheet, a free copy of which is available at www.hopecouples.com.

Intervention 22-1 Idea #1 for Preparing Couples to Forgive and Reconcile—Consider Wartime

War is not a time for forgiveness and reconciliation. Sure, certain acts are forgiven, but the big issues are not. Couples who are still at "war" with each other probably will not benefit much by engaging in forgiveness work that seeks to forgive the partner for most past offenses. That focus in therapy is almost certain to be unsuccessful and can poison future attempts to forgive. Even if forgiveness is successful early in therapy, partners might find that in the next ten minutes, there are new hurts to forgive. We might think that it is still a good thing to keep a short list of unforgiven or partially forgiven events. But the fact is, this will likely exhaust a warring couple so that when they get past the war and get ready to forgive, they will have lost confidence that forgiveness can be transformative.

For maximum benefit, the war needs to end first—or at least wind down in intensity. *Then,* an armistice is possible. That can be followed by working toward forgiveness. Couples should consider whether they feel that they are still at "war" or whether they are just having occasional "skirmishes." If the relationship is at "war," then stabilization work is needed before pursuing reconciliation.

To discuss in therapy. Have you ever tried to forgive and reconcile with someone in the midst of interpersonal war? How about after the war is over? Is your relationship at war, or do you just have an occasional "skirmish?" From your experience with family and friendship relationships, how do you know when a relationship is at "war?" (For more help with de-escalation and establishing relationship armistice, see Chapter 13 on conflict resolution.)

Intervention 22-2 Idea #2 for Preparing Couples to Reconcile—Why Forgive and Reconcile?

Wilhuf Tarkin (probably not a household name) is the fictional governor in *Star Wars* who commanded the Death Star (Episode 4). He was one of the most formidable villains in the franchise. He rules others by the fear of the use of force. Forgiveness needs to be motivated by positive relationship factors like love, compassion, empathy, or universal goodwill for others. Fear is a poor basis for forgiveness and undermines reconciliation.

To discuss in therapy. Have you ever been forced to forgive and reconcile with someone out of fear? What are you afraid of in your relationship now? How can reconciliation be motivated by positive emotions instead of fears?

Intervention 22-3 Idea #3 for Preparing Couples to Reconcile—Savor Good Forgiveness

Whiskey is one of the strongest but (some people, like Jen, think) most delicious drinks. It is powerful, requires aging, is valuable, and therefore is used judiciously. College students don't do "keggers" of fine whiskey!

Forgiveness is similar. An ounce of true forgiveness is better than a gallon of false forgiveness or even socially pressured forgiveness. Hollow forgiveness undermines reconciliation. True forgiveness with reconciliation requires time, care, and planning.

To discuss in therapy. Have you experienced a good, thoughtful, slow, caring forgiveness before? Either received or given? This discussion can lead to a discussion of the positive principles of emotional vs. decisional forgiveness and the REACH forgiveness model (discussed in Chapters 20 and 21). How can we reflect on how you have repaired and worked toward forgiveness as a couple so you can build trust to reconcile?

Discussion around Hurts (Step 2)

Discussions of hurts are emotional whirlwinds. They are rarely as orderly as we will present them here. But we are capturing the essence of two-party discussions of hurts and offenses.

Discussions about historical transgressions

To repair damage to the emotional bond, we best engage forgiveness (or some other technique for reducing the injustice gap) if we start with historical events that are outside the couple's relationship. The couple and therapist can reflect on historical patterns of pain, forgiveness, and reconciliation. Most couples locate these in their family of origin, past friendships, or past romantic partners. Releasing negative attributions about pain and finding more realistic complex attributions for causality can help couples. They can use communication skills practiced earlier in treatment to provide guardrails when discussing their histories of forgiveness and reconciliation.

After processing offenses from their past, they identify and process painful transgressions in their own relationship that continue to hinder their progress. Processing a historical transgression in their own relationship involves a soft (i.e., empathic, not finger-pointing) understanding of each partner's perspective. If lucky, they can figure out how to avoid similar future problems. They will need to take responsibility for their own mistakes, apologize, forgive their partner, and perhaps forgive themselves for their own part in the hurt.

Even if there aren't cosmic insights, processing old hurts can help release them from ruminative feedback, preventing the Zeigarnik effect—i.e., the power of unresolved questions.

Lumps and landmines in processing pain

When shoving regrettable incidents under the rug, the rug gets lumpy and can trip one up. Psychologically, when we have experienced something that still troubles us, we need to lift the corner of the metaphorical rug and sweep out the old dirt. Then, we can let it go and not have it trip us up later.

When couples are discussing past harms or conflicts, the most frequent mistake we see is that they continue to try to prove they were right originally. Unconsciously, they likely fantasize that their partner will give in and admit wrong-doing, and if not, the partner's failure to admit wrong-doing says that the partner is selfish, mean, and unforgiving.

They also might try to triangulate the therapist to be on their side. *If the therapist can be convinced,* they think, *the partner will have to knuckle under*. Instead, the therapist needs to redirect the couple to accept their different experiences of past events. Discuss giving the benefit of the doubt about the intent of their partner and explore any external stressors or negative cycles that contribute to the offense.

Detoxification of the Relationship—Readiness to Confess and Forgive (Step 3)

It is important to remember that readiness to hear a confession is an important stage in reconciliation. Readiness can be influenced by general stress and ability to cope. For example, a partner who was just laid off from work, got a new medical diagnosis, or realized their child suddenly dropped out of college may not have the resources to respond to a confession. Reconciliation may be delayed if either partner has high stress or difficulty coping.

A major way to detoxify a relationship is to give and receive a good account of their offense with a clear confession. This is a blurry line between discussing and detoxifying. For a discussion of transgressions to lead to detoxing, the offender, or perhaps both offenders, must make good accounts of their wrong-doings. Often, detox does not begin on the first good discussion that ends in confession. Maybe on the third or fourth. Not all partners will use confession to detoxify a relationship, but giving an account with a contrite confession helps remove some of the sting from the offense. Good confessions, which we will cover in the next chapter, end with hope that the person who was offended can forgive.

If we are pressed to decide when detoxing a relationship begins (although there probably is no practical use of such discernment), then responding to a request to forgive is where we would draw that arbitrary line. So, we will discuss detoxing the relationship by beginning with the response to a request to forgive. There are four ways people could respond:

1. refusing to forgive,
2. defining the offense as unforgivable,
3. agreeing to forgive (to decide and work toward emotional forgiveness),
4. delaying forgiveness by saying something like, "I can't decide. I need more time."

Devote to Living in Reconciliation (Step 4)

Most couples who are going through reconciliation need a strong commitment to the long-term efforts required of reconciliation. Movement is rarely linear. It is often characterized by stops, starts, setbacks, and struggles. Again, the stress-and-coping model of forgiveness can be helpful. Continuing the journey of reconciliation after major offenses, or many minor ones, can deplete resources. Practices and habits in the relationship that build the bond and counteract old offensive patterns are needed to give the couple their best chance at long-term forgiveness and reconciliation.

Conclusion

In this chapter, we have tried to give a broad overview of the Bridge to Reconciliation. That "bridge" is a metaphor to capture four steps in FREE. In the next three chapters, we give attention to each of the four steps.

Reference

Worthington, E. L., Jr. (2006). *Forgiveness and Reconciliation: Theory and Application*. Brunner-Routledge.

23 Making Decisions and Discussing Hurts

Discern What Can and Can't Be Redeemed

Problem:	Reconciliation requires a wise evaluation and open discussion of what can be redeemed.
Solution:	Good discussions with a therapist can clarify poor evaluations to move forward as a couple.

Most of the time, deciding whether to reconcile has been largely done by the time a couple reaches couple therapy. They have at least decided to give couple therapy a fighting chance. In the hope-focused couple approach (HFCA), the place to make decisions about reconciliation is in the assessment phase.

That does not mean the war is over. Obviously, many couples decide to discontinue efforts to reconcile mid-stream. They decide that their relationship is irredeemable. So, decisions are still necessary. As they begin the process, one hang-up for many couples is squabbles about what happened. Their memories of offensive events often differ, and this can be a roadblock to progress.

Provide Evidence That Memories Can Be Wrong

The therapist might encounter an argument in which both partners are absolutely convinced that they remember an event accurately. But do they?

It's frustrating when both partners insist that they remember an event accurately—especially if it's vital who's correct—and they are completely unwilling to admit any inaccuracy, to change, or to move on. This is the essence of a power struggle, of course, as we've come across many times. The real issue is not who's correct, but is who can say. However, we can't just throw our hands up and send them home. We must dislodge the roadblock. One way to do that is bring in a neutral authority—science (see Intervention 23-1).

DOI: 10.4324/9781003009382-28

Intervention 23-1 Consider Memory of Past Conflicts with an Analogy

First, the therapist might say, "I don't know which of you might be remembering most accurately, and unless there is a video of the event, it is probably not ever possible to find out. But it is possible that both of you are mostly right, but highly likely, according to research, that neither of you is 100 percent right. Are you interested in hearing what psychological science has to say about memory?"

Point 1: Virtually all memories are faulty. Long-term memory is not a mental video of the events. We actually re-create long-term memories every time we recall them, and those re-creations are affected by the context, by our mood, by our emotional state, and by what people say to us about the event. So, long-term memories are full of inaccuracies.

Point 2: Studies after the 9–11 attacks on the World Trade Center revealed some things about memory (Sharot et al., 2007). First, people in the Downtown Manhattan area, where the attacks occurred, reported different memories than did those in Midtown Manhattan. In Downtown, they reported more sounds and smells. In Midtown, they reported more big-picture scenarios and relied more on videos to fuel their memories. Memory tests against recorded footage showed that Downtowners actually missed more big-picture details. They relied on shared talk with others who went through it and supercharged emotions, but they didn't refer to objective videos. Memory for facts suffered. Midtowners didn't have moment-by-moment details, the sights, the sounds, the smells. But they were more accurate in big-picture details.

Second, people who lost loved ones in the attack were more emotional than were people in the same locale who did not lose a loved one. But both made exactly the same number of memory errors. However, the highly emotionally engaged people were more certain that their memories were correct.

The points for the therapist to make are (1) Most long-term memories are likely incorrect in details. (2) People remember their experience of an event fairly accurately but don't remember things they didn't experience. (3) How certain you are that you are correct is not a good predictor that you remember accurately. (4) Conclusion: better to be humble about the limits of accurate memory when we disagree about what happened in the past.

Provide Structures That Help Them Discuss

One way to structure discussions is to direct partners to see the impact of their own actions on their partner and take responsibility for that (see Intervention 23-2). This is especially true when processing hurts.

Intervention 23-2 It's Not Only What I Did, but What My Partner Perceived I Did

- First, assume that each will have a different view, which is generally correct.
- Second, they know that an apology (for the sake of apologizing or moving on) is meaningless. Meaningful apologies take responsibility for what they did, and also consider their own role in what the partner perceived.
- Third, therapists process with the couple what each person did, what they think the partner did, and how that affects the couple.
- Fourth, the speaker tells what happened and digs to reveal feelings about it. The listener works hard to empathize.
- Fifth, after a person understands what I did, what the partner thinks I did, and how it affected the partner, the person must take responsibility for what they did and how it affected what was perceived.
- Sixth, partners must put their desire to win behind what is good for the relationship and the partner.
- Seventh, partners can meaningfully express remorse and apologize (i.e., be vulnerable).

Yet another way to structure productive discussions around hurts is to coach partners on effective responding. We have organized numerous suggestions within Intervention 23-3.

Intervention 23-3 Psychoeducation about Processing Past Offenses

- Share how you felt.
- Share what you believe is your reality.
- Validate the other's reality.

- Agree with things you can agree to. "I heard you say. . . . I understood you to mean. . . ."
- Share experiences and memories that might be triggers. Share stories of what might have made these triggers for you. Triggers escalate the conflict. So, when precisely did you feel like the conflict became serious?
- Accept responsibility for your contributions to the argument. Do not comment on what you think your partner's contributions were.
  - What set you up for the fight?
  - What do you regret having done?
  - What other contributions did you made?
  - What are you apologizing for?
  - If you accept your partner's apology, say so directly.
  - If you don't accept it, what do you need before you would accept it?
- After both have done these, then seek to plan what each partner can do to lower the chance of this happening again.

Discussion can be structured by helping partners express themselves without causing negative reciprocity. Sometimes people have a hard time expressing their deep emotions when they are hurt. Dan Wile (1988) is a master therapist whose work has been used by couple therapists with different theoretical approaches. When couples have difficulty expressing emotions productively, or when they express only negative emotions, Wile uses Intervention 23-4. He speaks first for the partner he has the hardest time empathizing with.

Intervention 23-4 Dan Wile's (1988, 2008) Empathic Responding

This might be triggered when a speaker makes a hurtful emotional statement. Wile stops the interaction before the partner can respond in kind. He says that partners need to talk about their emotions, and he isn't trying to prevent that.

Wile says to the partner who made the hurtful statement, "Do you mind me speaking for you?"

If permission is given, he pulls a chair beside the partner and rephrases, removing the venom and also saying underlying feelings. Therapists add words of love, respect, care, admiration, and valuing.

Wile turns to partner he just "spoke for," "Did I get it close to right? Are there other things you'd like to add?"

Then, Wile switches and expresses empathy alongside the other partner.

Moving Toward Forgiveness and Reconciliation

Discussions of wrong-doing prepare the way for a couple to consider whether they want to forgive and reconcile. The lines between forgiveness and reconciliation are blurry for most couples who enter couple therapy intent on staying together. Researchers make distinctions between forgiveness, which is internal, and reconciliation, which is dyadic. But partners often communicate their forgiveness, which is technically part of reconciliation, but seen by partners as part of forgiveness. Reconciliation involves discussing wrongs, detoxifying the relationship of communication poisons, and finally promoting more devotion. But what is mere discussion? What is seeking to detoxify the relationship from past wrongs through promoting forgiveness? How do they use repair activities other than forgiveness? And don't apologizing, making amends, and forgiving also build devotion? There is a lot of overlap. As much as I (Ev) am a definitional purist in research, I don't sweat it with couples in therapy.

So, we are going to fill this part of the book with ideas to engage in the joint effort of forgiveness and reconciliation. We have discussed the REACH forgiveness model in Part 4. So, we won't repeat that. But we will discuss couple therapy activities that move them toward applying REACH forgiveness to forgive transgressions against them and to forgive themselves for the transgressions they inflicted on their partner. Forgiveness and reconciliation are embedded in the FREE intervention.

FREE is a free-standing intervention. But we've found that jumping right into it feels to some couples impersonal—like a "program" is being run on them instead of a personal attempt to help them. We want to avoid that kind of mechanistic interpretation in favor of a patient-centered approach to therapy. Thus, it helps to prepare couples for the FREE interventions. We offer three interventions (Interventions 23-5, 23-6, and 23-7) to prepare people for the FREE intervention proper. One uses empathy (23-5); a second, emotional softening (23-6); and the third, emotion regulation (23-7). We also offer a fourth intervention (Intervention 23-8) for preparation prior to FREE, one that addresses partners' questions.

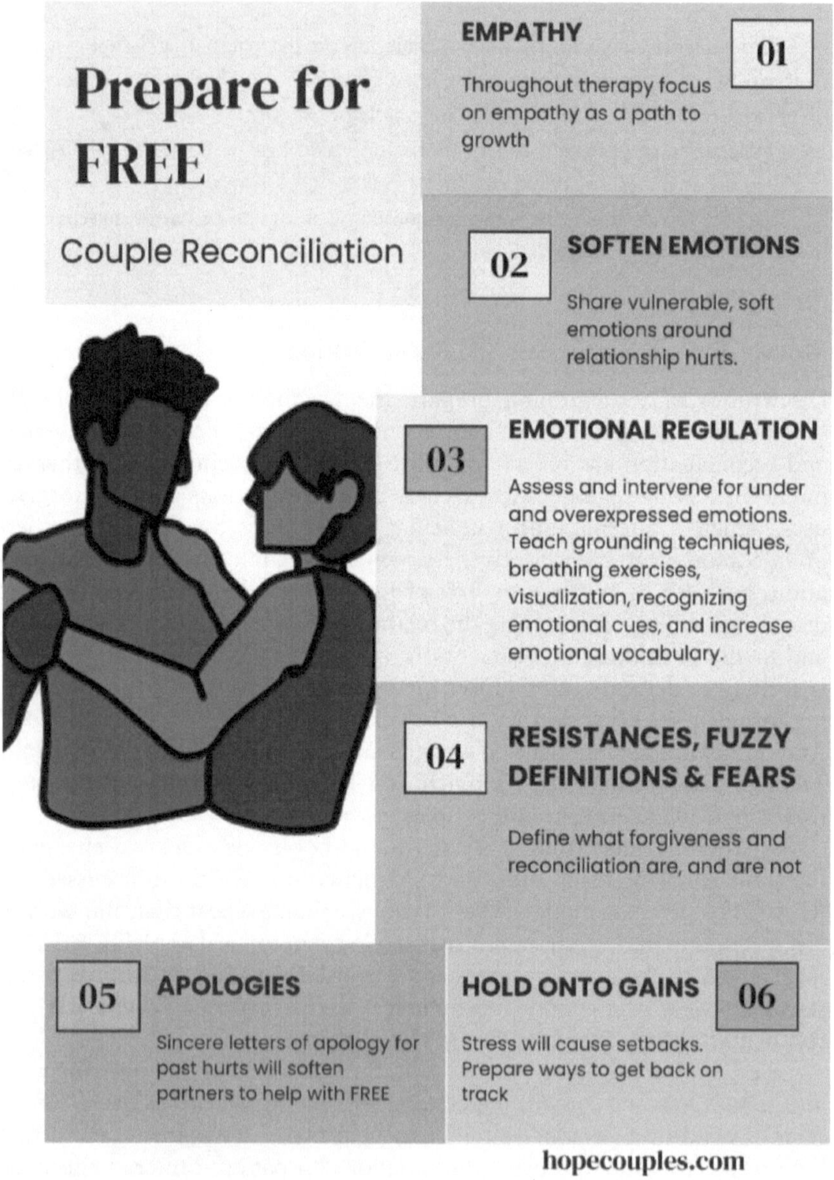

Figure 23-1 Prepare for FREE

Intervention 23-5 Preparing for Forgiveness and Reconciliation with Empathy

Therapists can direct couples toward empathic interactions in the weeks leading up to FREE. After all, the intervention is called "Forgiveness and Reconciling through Experiencing Empathy!" Fortunately, empathy is helpful across the techniques and goals of therapy. Empathy is great because it serves multiple goals. The couple improves communication or decreases conflict through empathy while, at the same time, they have had empathic experiences that help them navigate forgiveness and reconciliation. An empty-chair technique is especially helpful, using the chair to focus on hurts from parents or previous relationships to increase empathy for vulnerable spots in their partner's experience.

Intervention 23-6 Preparing for Forgiveness and Reconciliation with Emotional Softening

Prior to beginning work in FREE, the therapist hopes to promote emotional softening between the partners. Many couples enter therapy hard and defensive, attached to their fears more than each other. Softening is crucial in couple therapy (Furrow et al., 2012). Working on creating soft, vulnerable interactions through the bonding stage of therapy prepares partners to feel safer. If partners still feel alone, afraid, and helpless most of the time, they are likely not yet ready for FREE.

Intervention 23-7 Preparing for Forgiveness and Reconciliation through Regulating Emotions

Rumination can be a barrier to FREE and may need direct intervention. Emotional under- or over-expression may also need direct intervention. Physiological interventions, such as deep breathing or various grounding techniques, can assist partners in developing skills that will prepare them for difficult conversations that illicit anxiety. If partners can identify when emotional flooding starts, that will also allow them to call a time-out. Finding a safe place through visualization can help many clients. Under-expression of emotion may seem like it doesn't need assistance, but it might also represent numbing and avoidance. Under-expressers may need assistance expressing emotions, recognizing physical cues of emotions, and increasing emotional vocabulary.

Intervention 23-8 Address Resistance, Fuzzy Definitions, and Fears of Forgiveness

C.S. Lewis (1952) said, "Everyone says forgiveness is a lovely idea until they have something to forgive . . . And then, to mention the subject at all is to be greeted with howls of anger." Many people have experienced significant hurts around forgiveness and reconciliation. Small children are often forced to forgive without an adult understanding the bullying or mistreatment that has occurred. Domestic violence victims are sometimes encouraged to reconcile and return to dangerous home environments. The topic is not without its baggage. You don't know whether the bags are loaded unless you ask—openly and directly. Assume partners might resist FREE. Take time to explore their past experiences and beliefs. They might, for example, simply believe that forgiving requires that they give up all control. They hope that by not forgiving, they will keep their partner from re-engaging in hurtful actions. If it turns out your assumption is wrong and they are fine with forgiving and reconciling, great.

Help the partners decide how they define forgiveness. What is it and how is it different from reconciliation? The goal is to get the couple working together on forgiving and reconciling—not good definitional hygiene. Joint tasks like this predict positive change in relationships, so this is another "double-dip" activity for the couple. We recommend you try to get across a few concepts if possible: (1) forgiveness is inside their own skin individually and (2) there are two types of forgiveness, decisional and emotional.

Finally, encourage them to apply their definition to their lives. What would it mean to be more forgiving and reconcile as a couple? What specific activities are most likely to help them overcome fears and barriers to forgiveness and reconciliation?

Helping Partners Use the "Discuss" Part of FREE

When an offense has taken place, usually, the offended partner makes a request for an explanation of why the offending partner did so, called a *reproach*. We coach partners to make sensitive and empathy-driven reproaches. Instead of calling the offending partner names or seeking to humiliate the partner, give the partner the benefit of the doubt. The reproach should use I-language. Here's an example:

> When you told a joke at my expense last night, I was very hurt and I didn't feel supported. Usually, you are very sensitive and don't say things to get a laugh at my expense. So, I was surprised at what happened. I wonder whether you might share what was going on with you at that time?

When a partner has been gently and respectfully reproached, the offender can give one of four types of accounts of their behavior. They can *deny* that they did wrong (e.g., "I didn't do anything wrong" or "That was a harmless anecdote. You are just too sensitive."), which usually triggers an argument. They can *justify* what they did, which usually is done by blaming the partner in an I-only-did-it-because-you-hurt-me-first defensive retort. They also can *excuse* what they did. An excuse can be helpful because it tells extenuating reasons for the action (e.g., "I got thoroughly chewed out by my boss yesterday and my esteem was low, so I tried to get a laugh."). Or they can make a *confession* to the offense, which is also called making a *concession* to the correctness of the reproach. Generally, confessions keep people talking and able to resolve the issue.

Even if the offender believes that the reproach is incorrect, an empathic concession that states an understanding of why the partner might have perceived it as they did, keeps people talking. Confessions involve several parts. Apologies are vital because they indicate willingness to take responsibility, contrition, and care that values the partner. But, at another level, they are symbolic indications of willingness to be vulnerable and trust that the partner will not use the confession to psychologically injure the person apologizing.

When you approach a session that you intend to devote to discussions around forgiving, a good intervention is to ask partners to write letters of apology to their partner as homework (Intervention 23-9). This intervention was one of the first interventions created in FREE for couples (Worthington & DiBlasio, 1990) and has produced consistently good results with some dramatic moments in therapy. It works because it encourages partners—if they enter into the activity in good faith—to think about how they hurt their partners instead of their usual focus on how they were hurt. Couples often write meaningful, heart-felt apologies that can be tear-jerkers for couple and therapist alike. Even poorly written or rushed apology letters produce dramatic moments that reveal fears and struggles that are better addressed than left to fester underground.

Intervention 23-9 Write Letters of Apology as Homework

The first question is, are they ready to apologize and hear an apology? This intervention can help partners take responsibility for their own hurtful acts and move past the blame game.

For many couples, reviewing the principles of a good apology helps. These principles are described in Intervention 23-11: CONFESS Acronym.

After partners write letters of apology as homework, have partners read them to each other during the next session. This is usually an emotion-filled time that helps the couple. Even if it isn't helpful, the therapist is there to help partners work through poor apologies. Without pressure, discuss how helpful the apology was for each of them.

Apologies contain some risk; but they are usually worth the risk. They can lead to difficult conversations. (But, aw shucks, difficult conversations are what couple therapists are especially skilled at.) This intervention allows you to bring to bear your training in difficult dialogues for couples who still have fears and issues to work through. Trusting that the therapy process will be healing through apologies is key to staying grounded as a therapist. Be prepared for the ebb and flow of the impact of this emotion-filled intervention. For the couple that has a positive emotional session, you might even predict that they might sense fears arising again in the coming week, so they should watch for them and use emotion management skills to cope with fears or hurts.

Teach CONFESS as a Guide to a Good Account

Apologies are part of making a good confession. A good concession or confession admits to wrong-doing non-defensively. Then apologies are offered. Amends are offered and sometimes made. Then the victim might forgive the wrong-doer. There are many parts to a good confession. But before we teach an acronym to help cue people's memory of the steps to a good confession, some preliminary conversation with the couple is needed. Namely, the therapist needs to prepare the partners for different potential responses to an apology (see Intervention 23-10).

Intervention 23-10 Discuss Potential Responses to Being Asked to Forgive the Wrong-doer

Lay out the potential responses:

- No.
- I'll try, but it might take time especially for emotional healing.
- Yes, I forgive you. Socially acceptable words, but nonverbals convey that forgiveness is far from complete.
- Yes, I forgive you (believable and sincere).

Point out three apology-killers:

1 There will be pressure to say, "I forgive you." You don't have to say that. If a person confesses something, usually he or she has thought about it for a long time, but the other person might not even know about the wrong-doing. It might take quite a bit of time to get to the place where one is willing to forgive. Both partners need to affirm that, while it would be nice to hear an immediate "I forgive you," it is likely better to be more realistic that forgiveness usually takes time.
2 Try to avoid a flat "No." It ends conversation by driving a wedge between partners.
3 Besides responding to the request for forgiveness per se, discuss whether both people believe that amends are sufficient and that the offense might be prevented from recurring.

The therapist should teach the acronym CONFESS explicitly (Intervention 23-11), but the points may be drawn out by asking partners what would be needed to make a good confession, if they had wronged their partner. Then, the couple therapist can use CONFESS as a way to remind partners of what they likely already know, but likely do not have organized in their minds. Use clinical discernment to determine which approach to use with each couple.

Intervention 23-11 CONFESS Acronym

Therapist instructions: (1) Name the steps. (2) Model using it. (3) Discuss potential responses to being asked to forgive. (4) Ask each partner to try using it while looking at a printed copy of it. (5) Ask whether either (or both) would like to use CONFESS on a real event in which they feel they wronged the partner.

C = Confess without excuse. "I did x, and it was wrong" period.
O = Offer an apology believably, conveying regret, remorse, and sorrow at what you did.
N = Note the other's pain. Let the person you harmed know that you understand how much impact your wrong-doing had.
F = Forever value. "I value you and our relationship more than I value holding onto the mistaken view that I was completely right."
E = Equalize. Offer to make amends or, if necessary, pay it forward.
S = Say "Never again." State that you'll try not to harm the person that way again. In fact, you'll try not to hurt them in any way.
S = Seek forgiveness "Can you forgive me?"

There still might be many things partners need to discuss to ensure that the amends-making is sufficient (i.e., in the E-step) and that the offense or harm is not repeated (i.e., the first S-step).

There might be some sticking points in confessing wrong-doing that interrupt the flow and bog down the process. That is the nature of hurt feelings. They must be dealt with. First, confession might be tepid or inadequate. Some statements do not take responsibility for wrong-doing. They might convey that the offender didn't do anything wrong, as in "Sorry you feel that I hurt you (when in fact I didn't)." Some statements can be framed to hurt the partner. For example, "Sorry you are so overly sensitive." Some apologies do not convey regret and remorse; "Sorry I forgot our anniversary but I was overwhelmed at work." A second sticking point can be unwillingness to offer any, or a sufficient amount of, amends making. (A later sticking point is that the offender offers to make amends, but then never follows through.) A third sticking point can be how victims respond to being asked for forgiveness. There are many reasons that this can be a sticking point, such as believing that much restitution is needed prior to forgiving or being unwilling to forgive for principled reasons, including potential religious reasons. When CONFESS is used, it, and preparation for it, will require an entire session.

Conclusion

The discussion of the offense is, in some ways, not yet over. We don't know how the partner will respond to the request of the offender for forgiveness. However, some responses can lead to substantial healing in the relationship. So, we are moving the victim's response to a request for forgiveness to the next chapter, on detoxification of the relationship.

References

Furrow, J. L., Edwards, S. A., Choi, Y., & Bradley, B. (2012). Therapist presence in emotionally focused couple therapy blamer softening events: Promoting change through emotional experience. *Journal of Marital and Family Therapy*, *38*(s1), 39–49. https://doi.org/10.1111/j.1752-0606.2012.00293.x

Lewis, C. S. (1952). *A Preface to Paradise Lost*. HarperOne.

Sharot, T., Martorella, E. A., Delgado, M. R., & Phelps, E. A. (2007). How personal experience modulates the neural circuitry of memories of September 11. *PNAS Proceedings of the National Academy of Sciences of the United States of America, 104*(1), 389–394. https://doi.org/10.1073/pnas.0609230103

Wile, D. B. (1988). In search of the curative principle in couples therapy. *Journal of Family Psychology*, 2(1), 24–27. https://doi.org/10.1037/h0080486

Wile, D. B. (2008). *After the Honeymoon: How Conflict can Improve your Relationship*. Daniel Wile.

Worthington, E. L., Jr., & DiBlasio, F. A. (1990). Promoting mutual forgiveness within the fractured relationship. *Psychotherapy, 27*, 219–223.

24 Repairing Damage to the Relationship

Fix What Can Be Fixed

Problem:	The injustice gap in couples can be severe.
Solution:	Learn ways to love and live with unresolvable problems.

The troubled relationship has inevitably accumulated some poisons. Many of those poisons center on particular harms or offenses that are not fully forgiven. In this chapter, we examine how couples can discuss harms soon after they occur without adding to the toxins. Partners often need to discuss how to change their injustice gaps; many toxins in the relationship may be due to accumulated toxins from patterns that might have gone on for years. So, we cover how to help couples recover from long-term accumulation of toxins. Finally, we consider how to cope with irresolvable strains on the relationship.

Repairing Deeply Wounding Offenses and Hurts by Forgiving Them

A partner who has deep wounds and hurts from the relationship wants to be protected. Protection activities often warp the relationship. To feel protected, partners might withdraw often, protest loudly, complain to friends to elicit support, or numb themselves with bad habits. Those protective actions are understandable, but they create a stable, unhealthy system that protects but harms healthy connection. Part of detoxifying the relationship is communicating around one's request for forgiveness. We named some ways to respond to such requests in the previous chapter. We expand on them below.

Partners are in a mutual dance once a transgression has been experienced. We considered the offender in Chapter 23. We now examine the

DOI: 10.4324/9781003009382-29

person hurt or offended. Before we do, however, we recall that forgiveness is a choice, so partners do not have to forgive. But when a person makes a sincere and contrite confession and asks for or begs for forgiveness, the person is making himself or herself vulnerable. The person offended has several possible responses to the offender.

Refusal to forgive

If that vulnerability is trampled on by the victim not seeming to give even consideration to forgiving—or considering it but flatly refusing to forgive—that is not a good sign for the future of the relationship. Almost as discouraging for the future of the relationship is "conditional" forgiveness. Conditional forgiveness is to say that one will forgive if certain conditions are met. Often, in troubled relationships, those conditions are restrictive, oppressive, coercive, or manipulative. The meeting of vulnerability with coercion or manipulation is likely to produce resentment and will almost inevitably lead the manipulated person to rebel and fight against such control.

Forgiveness is a choice, of course, so an offended partner does not have to forgive no matter how eloquent and heart-rending the plea. As a therapist, you can recognize aloud that the offended partner seems disinclined to forgive. Instead of pushing for forgiveness, you can advise using alternatives to forgiveness to deal with injustice.

Immediate forgiveness

If the person who was deeply offended says, "Of course, I forgive you," both the therapist and partner might distrust that statement. Not that the forgiver is deceitful (though that has certainly happened), but a glib offer of forgiveness seems to indicate a naïve or non-self-aware forgiver.

This puts you in a bind. You don't want to insult the forgiver by implying that you don't believe him or her. But you also don't want to accept this statement at face value when a lot of emotional negativity lurks underneath the surface.

It is wise to ask what the forgiver means by the statement of forgiveness. This could indicate that the forgiver has thought about it long and hard and made a sincere decision to forgive. But, it could also indicate that unrealistic expectations, that are a sure set-up for failure, are held or that the forgiver is implying that it's open season to offend and (by tit-for-tat) all transgressions will be swept under the rug. It could mean that they expect absolutely flawless future behavior from the contrite partner, and any deviation from perfection will be considered grounds for some unspoken dire consequences to the relationship. Sometimes, partners are quick to jump to immediate forgiveness as a signal that they "just want this pain to be over." This is especially true if the offense is causing relational storming and dysregulation. Reflecting on both their desire to move forward and find peace together can build motivation toward reconciliation. The point is, if you don't ask, you don't know. So, if the partner does not ask, then ask the forgiver what he or she means by the generous forgiveness that is seemingly offered.

You might find, on occasion, that someone is deeply aware of the gravity of the offense and the hurt that both partners have suffered. They courageously want to forgive anyway and are stating that decision (even though little emotional forgiveness has been experienced). Even there, it's helpful to ponder that there might be "parts of self" that don't feel forgiving, are angry, or might fall back on unforgiveness easily. A more complex understanding of forgiveness can help partners as they work through the complexities of repairing offenses.

I can't forgive yet

Or perhaps the offended partner will say the equivalent of, "I have decided to forgive you, but I still feel emotional unforgiveness." Naturally, almost no couple will use those words but will be saying essentially the same thing. They might say, "I do forgive you, but I'm not over this yet. It still feels raw." Or they might say, "I do forgive you, but that doesn't mean we are back to where we were before you had the affair."

Communicating forgiveness in response to a request to forgive is rarely as simple as it sounds

There are undertones, expectations, and hidden agendas galore that need exploration. The size of the injustice gap often drives whether the offended partner will decide to forgive. The wrong-doing partner has options to reduce the size of the injustice gap as we have described. But in communicating about the injustice gap and forgiveness, making amends looms large.

Communication Around the Injustice Gap

You can promote communication that ultimately leads to a smaller injustice gap. One way the injustice gap can be transcended is for the offended partner to forgive. But at first, you'll want to promote more general communication about closing the injustice gap. Intervention 24-1 helps people see the partner's perception of the injustice gap more accurately.

Intervention 24-1 Scaling the Injustice Gap

Therapists can intervene with the couple by having them scale the injustice gap from 0 to 10 in severity. Jen has had good experiences with this. Here's how she uses it.

- Have the partners each pick a recent offense.
- They rate the injustice gap of both offenses: the one they caused and the one they received. (It's amazing how often the one they caused is rated a 1–3, while the received offense is rated 4–7+.)
- Ask partners to interpret why this pattern was seen.
- Suggest that the pattern is due to physically experiencing the pain received, but not the pain they inflicted.

Partners' realizations that they are under-estimating the amount they are hurting their partner can affect both partners. It can create empathy. But sometimes partners can get defensive. One way to short-circuit defensiveness is, if you know you are going to use this intervention prior to the session, then write your prediction ahead of time. That way, it appears more like a general finding that feels less like the partner just mis-estimated on a particular hurt.

Reflect on patterns of amends

As people confess wrong-doing, offering to make amends usually arises. It is helpful to get partners to discuss their history of making amends around this or similar offenses in the past. You can ask, "What has worked for you in the past?" If you need suggestions to prompt their discussion, here are some. Amends-making can include things like:

- presents (which usually comes to mind quickly), but on a more relational level . . .
- stating commitments to the relationship,
- words of love and affection,
- grand romantic gestures,
- increased work on the relationship, or
- forgiveness.

Illuminating patterns of injury and repair across their relationships—both as a couple and in other important relationships—can help partners see where they need to let go of hostility or negative affect and make and accept repair attempts.

Detox to Repair Accumulated Damage to the Emotional Bond

Not all relationship detoxification is around specific hurts or offenses. Some happen because hurts build up over time and eventually become aggravating. Some seemingly irreconcilable issues become perennial (e.g., one person can't stand the in-laws and yet visits are expected, or differences in spending versus saving don't seem resolvable). After a while, because of the long-term patterns, the quality of the relationship deteriorates. Perhaps couple therapy has helped, but there might be abiding frustrating topics that will far outlive couple therapy and will continue to poison the relationship unless they are dealt with. Perhaps you can't solve all of these problems in couple therapy, but you might be able to help partners handle these after therapy is over.

What to do about the four horsemen of the apocalypse

Gottman (1993) showed that as relationships disintegrate, they pass through four "stages," with the appropriate caution that no relationship follows a lock-step progression through the stages. So, dealing with the dissolution of relationships is similarly not a formula. Rather, we provide a general guideline as a first line of therapy for dissolving relationships. First, we will want to get the emotional flooding under control. Second, we will want to repair the damage.

Respond quickly to emotional floods

What couples do after the flood storm hits and clears the yard is important. Couple hurts and offenses are one storm, but they can bring up old hurts and create worst storms than the immediate one. Amanda Ripley (2022) described the Hatfield and McCoy feud in her book, *High Conflict*. The 80-year feud started over (wait for it) a pig. McCoy noticed a pig he thought belonged to him in Hatfield's pig pen. He sued. In a trial with six Hatfields and six McCoys in the jury box, McCoy lost his suit. Ten years later, a witness at the trial provoked three McCoy boys, who beat the witness to death. A seemingly resolved dispute, ten years later, triggered the murder and the feud.

When a couple has an emotional flood, how they attempt to reduce the flood and repair things is important. They don't want a seeming resolution (like the Hatfield—McCoy trial verdict) that leaves an undercurrent of resentment that can flare up later.

Gottman's (1993) four horsemen of the apocalypse is a guide map to untreated relationship storms: Criticism and defensiveness, then contempt and stonewalling. Therapists can help couples create realistic responses to relationship collapse. In the immediate aftermath of a flare up, Intervention 24-2 shows how therapists can help partners respond quickly to criticism non-defensively when it occurs in session.

Intervention 24-2 Responding to Criticism Non-Defensively (In Session)

Suggest that the partners practice a simple three-step way of responding to criticism (or to felt criticism) without defensiveness. I feel, see, and ask is the phrase to remember.

Step 1: I feel

Label the emotions. Example: "I'm feeling defensive and a little hurt right now."

Step 2: I see it this way

Describe the situation that triggered the feeling. Try not to blame. Say *what* each partner saw from their perspective, not who. If you must say who, try to treat it as an impartial observation rather than something the partner did that was wrong. Example: "I forgot and asked you three times what you were doing after breakfast. Sorry. When you sighed, I got defensive because I felt I had done wrong."

Step 3: I ask

Say what is needed from the partner to feel better. Example: "I ask whether you can try not to sigh when I exasperate you. Can you just patiently answer my question?" If possible, add an "I'll try" statement, like "I'll try not to frustrate you as often."

Responding quickly can often reduce flooding because the emotional waters are diverted to productive use. But sometimes, the emotional flood will have set in motion unresolved past emotions. Those can rise quickly and trigger hot conflict. This is especially true when relationships are disintegrating. In failing relationships, partners will usually rehearse the many past emotional flare-ups. So, when partners anticipate talking about the relationship, arousal takes place, bubbling up from past and present hurts. Both partners quickly get aroused. Recall that, generally, freezing, fleeing, or fighting come about because people feel emotionally flooded. So, usually before much discussion can occur, the couple needs to reduce emotional flooding.

Some rare couples can calm themselves in the midst of a conflict—especially if the conflict is not hugely emotionally engaging. But most couples might want to have a cool-down period—at least briefly—after the topic of "we need to talk" is broached.

Broach the topic softly

So, the conversation might start with one partner saying, "We seem to be having more trouble with the relationship lately. I think we need to talk and see what we might do to get back on track. When would be a good time to talk?"

Schedule the talk

The other might agree that talk is needed but might not be ready at the present. The one suggesting the talk has likely been thinking about it, but the other person feels that the issue has been "sprung" on them. So, ideally, the one proposing the talk might suggest that talking in 30 minutes or the following morning might be a good time. This provides a cool-down period that is not simply an adrenaline-fueled reaction to the "we-need-to-talk" opening. During that period, ideally, each will self-soothe and think of major issues that need discussion.

Self-soothe

Partners differ in how they self-soothe, and the internet has hundreds of suggestions for self-soothing if clients need ideas. Often, it is by distraction or calming, but it does not involve planning the next attack. Vigorous exercise works for some, but angry activity, like slamming a pickleball against the side of the house, will keep the body activated and can lead to aggression when the discussion is resumed. After the stated time period, the partners will re-engage, perhaps over a cup of tea or coffee, and discuss the difference.

The focus of the discussion

This is not a discussion about a particular wrong. This is a strategy session done with the idea of identifying the state of the relationship and then trying to "move the needle" to a better state. The tendency—because we are all human—is to assume that the way to move the needle is for the other person to change. The best results will be obtained, though, if each person accepts responsibility for his or her part and offers ways that he or she might change.

The strategy

The discussion will have a strategy (a grand plan) and tactics (ways that the strategy is put into practice). The strategy might be to identify (1) what stage of the four horsemen the relationship is functioning at and (2) ways that the relationship can move up a level. That is, if the partners are in Gottman's war or contempt stage, they usually are thinking about the stable personality "flaws" in the partner or aspects of the relationship not amenable to change. So, how can they move back to issue-oriented conflicts that might still be characterized by criticism and defensiveness? At least there is hope that change can occur. If they are enmeshed in criticism and defensiveness, they might try to figure out how to cut down the frequency. One way is to use the solution-focused therapy idea of just moving the needle a small amount rather than setting a likely unachievable goal of eliminating all criticism and defensiveness.

The tactics

The tactics used by each will test whether the partners can put into effect the things they learned in therapy about resolving conflict and communicating. They will start with a gentle start-up rather than a harsh start-up (Lisitsa, 2023), realizing that the first three minutes of a discussion can predict how the discussion might progress until it is completed. Gottman has shown that the first three minutes of a conflict discussion can predict the status of the relationship up to six years in the future, so a gentle start-up is important. Then, perhaps they will use the LOVE acronym (L=Listen and repeat; O=Observe your effects; V=Value your partner; E=Evaluate both people's interests behind positions) or a speaker–listener method.

Working with Unresolvable Complicating Problems

Couples deal with different complicating problems. Those are usually chronic. Some, like many addictive behaviors are largely due to one partner's choices. But the problems might be no one's fault, and they might not be fixable. For example, these might include such things as children with severe problems, prescription-drug dependence or addiction by one partner, chronic self-control issues that affect the health of an individual or provide a threat to the well-being of the relationship, acute mental health disorders, chronic personality disorders by one partner, needed care for elderly parents when insufficient funds are available for a care facility, a toxic work environment by one (or both) partners, and the experience of chronic pain or illness in one of both partners.

The key to dealing with unresolvable problems is admitting that there might be no good solution and that the problem is jeopardizing the relationship. This is not an invitation to helplessness, hopelessness, powerlessness, and depression. There are things that can be done to cope with the situation and the stresses it places on the relationship, even though there might be no solution to the problem per se. In almost all of the complicated problems above, partners must work together, and sacrifices will be needed by one partner more than the other partner.

Ev got some good advice along these lines on his wedding day. When Ev and Kirby married, Ev was in the Navy stationed near San Francisco, and Kirby, having just completed a master's degree at the Ohio State University, was at her parents' home in South Florida. Ev's roomies took him to dinner to celebrate his all-night flight to Florida for the wedding. And, as luck would have it, they were robbed in the restaurant. Well-equipped with adrenaline, Ev then got on the midnight flight to Florida and attempted to memorize his vows. The stress of impending marriage plus robbery was too much, as he found out during the service as he said his vows. The pastor had to prompt him on every phrase.

Ev: I, uh . . . (awkward pause as people look at him).
Pastor: Ev?
Ev: Right. I, Ev, . . . (awkward pause)

You get the idea. Anyway, before the ceremony started with that unforgettable moment, Ev was sitting on the couch in Kirby's living room. Her father, a six-four, four-sport college athlete and current principal of a high school, was standing (benignly, we're sure) over Ev.

"Marriage is not a 50–50 proposition," he said.

Ev swallowed his bubble gum. "Uh, gulp, no, sir. I mean, yes, sir, I mean. . . .

"It's a 100–100 proposition! There will be times in your marriage when you give 100 percent and get nothing. There will be other times when you give nothing and get 100 percent from Kirby. *Don't keep score.*"

Those difficult situations are the times when one partner is called on to give quite a bit more than he or she gets—what the interdependence theorists call diagnostic situations. They challenge partners to show whether they are fundamentally for themselves, or whether they will value their relationship and their partner enough to put aside self-interest—at least for a while. It is those very situations that challenge and yet often solidify the relationship. Those are times that can be gifted to the relationship if people are serious about their vows—for better or for worse, for richer or poorer, in sickness and in health—which were said aloud in public (even if they had to be prompted at every turn by a patient pastor).

It is possible for the couple therapist to facilitate partners accepting what cannot be changed and yet finding ways that partners might cope with the intractable situation. Here are some pieces of advice to therapists (Intervention 24-3).

Intervention 24-3 Principles to Address Unresolvable Problems

Here are three pieces of advice for therapists working with couples with unresolvable problems.

- Help the couple with de-flooding skills or regulating emotions. Both partners need this skill, even if they ultimately divorce.
- Reflect with them (sometimes individually) on the nature of their commitment. Some recently dating couples, still supercharged by love hormones, will engage in high sacrifice for a partner. Couples with high commitments like marriage, children, or years of a life together shouldn't be discouraged from making their own choices to engage in courageous sacrifice. Sometimes, as therapists, we are rankled when we see a needy client sacrificing on behalf of their relationship. Rankled or not, we know that familial needs might take priority over individual needs, and we can help the client make the courageous choice.
- Talk honestly with the couple about how "the problem" will make this uneven between them—at least for a time. This is especially difficult in Western friendship-based relationships that feel like they ought to be 50–50 at all times. But the person who is helping should reflect back on the 100–100 principle of stable romantic relationships that were conveyed so forcefully by Ev's father-in-law. The person with the problem should ponder ways to use their own strengths to give what they can to the relationship.

Boundaries around high conflict, unhealthy, or dangerous interactions will need special attention. Partners will need to learn to take breaks, not fix everything for the person with a problem, and not be emotionally enmeshed and overfocused on the problem.

Conclusion

Detoxifying the relationship is sometimes a problem that can be interminable if a chronic condition exists that cannot be solved but must just be coped with. At other times, detoxing the relationship can lead to a strategic conversation about how to arrest the downslide of a failing relationship. At other times, detoxing can be relegated to simply getting past a deeply wounding transgression.

Each type of detox situation has its own challenges and rewards. All seem to boil down, though, to valuing the partner and the relationship, to working on and putting continual energy into bettering the relationship, and to having a deep faith in the partner and the relationship. In a phrase, to faith, work, and love.

References

Gottman, J. M. (1993). A theory of marital dissolution and stability: Families in transition. *Journal of Family Psychology*, 7(1), 57–75.

Lisitsa, E. (2023). *How to Fight Smart: Soften your Start Up*. Retrieved September 7, 2023, from https://www.gottman.com/blog/softening-startup/

Ripley, A. (2022). *High Conflict: Why We Get Trapped and How We Get Out*. Simon and Schuster.

25 Rebuilding Devotion with FREE

Create New Structures to Replace Missing Ones

Problem:	Rebuilding damaged relationships requires intentional work.
Solution:	Use FREE principles to rebuild trust and positive relationship bond.

One of the most moving reconciliation stories we know came after World War II. On November 14, 1940, the most concentrated attack on any British city occurred. Coventry was essentially razed. Over 500 Luftwaffe bombers raided Coventry for 11 hours. The St. Michael's Church was destroyed—the only British cathedral destroyed in the war. More than 43,000 homes were destroyed or damaged. The death toll was over 500 people.

The Allied forces retaliated—in spades. On February 13–15, 1945, the Allied bombing of Dresden became one of the most controversial bombings of the war. Over 800 bombers attacked on February 13 and set off a firestorm. The next day, US bombers dropped bombs. On February 15, 210 additional bombers dropped bombs. Altogether, the three bombings killed over 25,000 people and destroyed over 73,000 homes. A historic cathedral, Frauenkirche (Cathedral of Our Lady), was also destroyed.

Neither city was of strategic importance. Because a major religious center was destroyed at each location, the bombings became symbols of religious desecration, which is especially hard to forgive. Yet, both the Coventry Chapel and Frauenkirche were rebuilt after the war ended. Both received financial support from around the world. In a twist, Coventry received substantial support from West Germany, and Dresden received substantial support from the British Dresden Trust. The pair of cathedrals—symbols of desecration—became symbols of reconciliation after serious and morally deficient attempts to destroy the other. Both rebuilt cathedrals contain not only structurally sound walls, floors, support beams, and ceilings, but also religious symbols of reconciliation.

DOI: 10.4324/9781003009382-30

This can be a metaphor for reconciling and rebuilding marriage, especially after the partners might have tried to destroy each other and things they held sacred. Such sacred objects might be the marriage itself, the family, or even each partner's identity. Learning about this historic event could speak cogently to couples who have felt like they have been at war (see Intervention 25-1).

Intervention 25-1 For Marriage-War Survivors, Read about Coventry and Dresden

If the therapist deems it appropriate, ask formerly "warring" partners to research the Coventry and Dresden bombings, reconstruction, and reconciliation efforts online. Discuss their findings and ask whether they wanted to rebuild the structures of their relationship.

In devotion, this last part of reconciliation, we seek to help partners solidify the gains they have made in couple therapy by promoting positive devotion to each other. All previous parts of reconciliation—decisions, discussion, and detoxification—have focused on repairing problems. Now, partners build renewed devotion, which is more about growing new structures or renewing the functioning of structures that had been damaged earlier. In devotion, partners maintain and increase functionality. The major principles for increasing devotion and maintaining gains are:

1 recognize partner and couple behaviors that maintain or accelerate changes,
2 reinforce valuing love by repetition or by intervening in a new way,
3 motivate the couple to continue to pour effort into the relationship,
4 avoid or prevent pressures that might propel partners back into problems, and
5 use preventive maintenance to avoid future problems.

In this chapter, we discuss two topics. We seek to solidify new patterns partners built during therapy. We also look to the future and ask partners to recommit to the core strategic principles—love, work, and faith.

Solidify New Patterns of Relating to Each Other

As couples near the end of the bridge to reconciliation, they have almost completed couple therapy. They are past stages of remoralization and remediation. Now they need to firm up gains of therapy into new patterns. New patterns of emotions and behavior can help restore trust.

Positive emotions are one key to building devotion. Gratitude can powerfully build trust. Gratitude interventions are good early in treatment to build momentum and hope for change, but they also serve the end of treatment by building devotion. In Intervention 25-2, we suggest several evidence-based gratitude interventions.

Intervention 25-2 Increase Devotion through Gratitude Interventions

Partners can:

- Write letters of gratitude focused on their partner; religious couples can write a letter to God as a prayer to engage their spiritual values.
- Read positive letters in therapy to bring positive emotions into the session.
- Use creativity to make a work of art or craft (i.e., plant a tree, paint a picture, or adopt a pet with a name that means grateful, like the African name Shakira) that expresses gratitude for their partner and relationship.
- Host celebrations; public expressions of gratitude can be especially positive flooding experiences.

Recommit to Love, Work, and Faith

Many practical ways to solidify new patterns of behavior involve re-committing to the principles that we have stressed in this book—promoting love, work, and faith—but this time without therapist oversight. Partners must monitor themselves, without critiquing the partner, on whether they are valuing their partner and not devaluing the partner (i.e., love), investing enough energy into keeping the relationship moving positively (i.e., work), and having faith in the partner, the relationship, and the self (i.e., faith). Partners can take this commitment seriously and change their own behavior when they feel that they are not performing up to their current standards.

If couples are able to do these things successfully, they become, in the ideal, something like what the Gottman couple therapy system calls a master of relationships, which is characterized by friendship. Importantly, this is an ideal. Of course, not all couples would agree that this is their ideal. In conflict, masters of relationships can repair damage.

Everyone gets emotionally flooded and negative at times. Conflicts happen. Masters of relationships, however, calm down, step back, and get out of the conflict-dominated system. They can say something like, "I'm sorry. That did not come out like I intended it to. Can we talk about this again?"

Ev's 2006 Blue Prius has over 250,000 miles on it and has not needed any repair beyond preventive maintenance. Preventive maintenance is important to keeping any engine running smoothly. Of course, as amazingly complicated as automotive technology is, a long-term romantic relationship is an order of magnitude more complicated. Still, the principles of preventive maintenance can serve as a guide for partners who are about to leave therapy. The general categories of preventive maintenance are (1) provide sufficient lubrication to keep friction and heat to a low ebb, (2) keep the engine clean so no foreign matter clogs up and interferes with functioning, (3) keep the machine tuned up, (4) make regular checks on functioning, and (5) replace damaged or worn parts that are no longer functioning as they are supposed to.

Friction is due to conflict. Conflict occurs more frequently when partners become pressured and "short" with each other. It also occurs when partners feel a loss of freedom, autonomy, or intimacy. Keeping the intimacy–distance–co-action balanced maintains smooth functioning. Big changes in time commitments, health, or stressors can disrupt that balance and introduce conflicts. Friction in relationships is often kept low through social lubrication. That means using positive, valuing, loving behaviors. This can involve spending pleasurable time together, having sex regularly, doing special things occasionally, like eating out at special places or going to movies or plays. But relational friction is also minimized by taking care of little problems before they become big problems.

Couples in the maintenance stage refuse to allow impurities back into their relationship—such as allowing valuing love to wane, getting distracted so that work on the relationship declines, and losing faith in their partner's work on the relationship. Impurities could be an unhealthy attachment to other relationships and over-investment in jobs, hobbies, or friends. It also could involve one (or both) partners changing their behaviors to insert unfavorable behaviors or eliminate favorable behaviors.

Engaging in periodic check-ups might be the most difficult part of preventive maintenance. Once finished with therapy sessions, it is easy to fall into a routine and forget preventive maintenance. In fact, intentionally re-evaluating the relationship might cause anxiety if they find the problems exist. States know this, so they mandate annual state inspections of autos. Use Intervention 25-3 to interest couples in regular check-ups. Even if they don't take you up on it, it can be a reminder to keep promoting faith, work, and love in their relationship.

Intervention 25-3 Motivate Couples to Use Regular Checks on Functioning

We can aid memory by tying a marital check-up to the anniversary. Or, perhaps partners take an annual trip to Disney World or camp in the mountains. They could tie their scheduled trip to their relationship check-up.

The check-up does not have to be extensive, but it should be as comprehensive across the relationship as possible. We have provided a set of suggested questions (see Intervention 25-4) to reflect on, perhaps answer in writing and then discuss. These questions reinforce the primacy of a close emotional bond and use the categories of love, work, and faith to evaluate the relationship. Provide this set of questions directly to the couple as therapy winds down.

Intervention 25-4 Discuss Annual Relationship Check-up Questions

Reflect on, and write answers to, the following thought questions. Schedule a time when you can discuss these with your partner. Tying this evaluation and discussion to regularly scheduled events within your relationship will help you.

Emotional Bond

The cause of a good relationship is a strong emotional bond. That is, this is the closeness that I feel to my partner and my partner feels to me.

- Do we feel we have a strong emotional bond that we are each satisfied with? Do we both agree on this?
- If you feel that more (or less) emotional connection is needed, can you suggest one or two things that you could do differently to move the relationship where you would be more comfortable, your partner would be more comfortable, and both would agree more?

Love

Love is valuing your partner and not devaluing your partner.

- How do you feel you are doing in that regard? Could you do anything different? (Your task here is not to critique your partner but to ponder how you could value your partner more.)

Work

- Are you putting enough time into your relationship? Is it good-quality time? Or is it just "spending time" without promoting a good relationship?
- If you think you could put more effort into the relationship, note at least two different things you could do to make things better.

Faith

- Faith in the relationship is the sense that you believe the relationship is working well and is resilient to challenges. How do you evaluate your faith in your relationship?
- Faith in yourself as a relationship partner is your sense that you are able to count on yourself to put energy into the relationship and give it enough importance in your life that it really matters. How do you evaluate the faith you have in yourself as a relationship partner?
- Faith in your partner is a sense that you can trust your partner. Do you believe you can trust your partner? In what areas?

Couples can use the CARE measure (Worthington et al., 1997) to help identify strengths or areas to focus on. The measure uses the same categories that we have emphasized throughout therapy.

Intervention 25-5 Use the CARE Measure to Have Couples Self-Evaluate the Relationship

The measure can be found at hopecouples.com in the assessments section. It asks about seven topics: (a) communication, (b) resolution of differences, (c) freedom from blaming the partner when things go wrong, (d) willingness to admit to having hurt the partner and to ask the partner for forgiveness, (e) ability to forgive the partner after a hurt, (f) intimacy, and (g) commitment to the partner for the long term. The 7-point response options range from couldn't be worse (1), terrible, bad, not bad/ not good, good, great, and couldn't be better (7), so the scores range from 7 to 49. Happy couples had a mean of 38 and SD = 7. Thus, 2/3 of the couples scored between 31 and 45. About 95 percent of the couples scored between 22 and 49. You can tell couples these ranges to help them interpret their own scores.

Couple therapy has one of the highest rates of recidivism (Ripley et al., 2021). Also, success rates are lower than therapy for all problems except addiction. In our own research of the hope-focused couple approach (HFCA), we found that around 30 percent of couples do not cross the threshold into the "non-clinical" rating after completing a course of couple therapy. Some regress after couple therapy ends. Yes, we are discouraged with those statistics, but take solace because they are similar to virtually all approaches to couple therapy.

Replace parts that are potentially problem-causing. In a car, we don't wait until the oil sump is empty to add oil or the oil has become degraded to change it. We monitor the oil level and time since last oil change, and we replace the oil before red lights go on. Similarly, in our relationships, we need to replace potentially problematic patterns of emotional floods, dysregulated behaviors, or detachment before they become problems. If one partner sees that they aren't spending as much time together as previously or that the type of activities has changed ("We don't have those long talks like we did last year."), the partner can bring the issue up for discussion.

You can use this auto preventive maintenance analogy in termination sessions to alert couples to post-therapy monitoring. And you can invite them to phone you for early assessment or intervention when needed.

Conclusion

Building renewed devotion into a relationship is not simple. The focus has been on repair throughout almost all of couple therapy, so it often seems like a disjointed shift when couple therapy moves to re-establishing positive functional relationships. Yet, that is a vital task in restoring the relationship that must continue even after therapy is done.

References

Ripley, J., Solfelt, L., Ord, A., Garthe, R. C., Worthington, E. L., Jr., & Channing, T. (2021). Short- and long-term outcomes of hope-focused couple therapy. *Spirituality in Clinical Practice*. Advance online publication. https://doi.org/10.1037/scp0000286

Worthington, E. L., Jr., Hight, T. L., Ripley, J. S., Perrone, K. M., Kurusu, T. A., & Jones, D. R. (1997). Strategic hope-focused relationship-enrichment counseling with individual couples. *Journal of Counseling Psychology, 44*, 381–389.

Part 6

Reforging Trust

26 Reforging Trust

Let Couples Know That It Takes Longer Than They Think It Will

Problem:	Trust is easily lost, and hard to regain for couples.
Solution:	Understand the process of trust-building and engage the couple in efforts to be trustworthy and trusting.

The couple was making progress in therapy. They had been trapped in a cycle where he was overstressed, emotionally reactive, inappropriately angry, and occasionally drinking too much. His primary goal was to be left in peace. She was critical, withdrawn, fearful, and unable to state her needs clearly and kindly. Her primary goal was to have a deeply loving, swoon-worthy, and kindly marriage relationship.

After 18 sessions, he had stopped drinking when they fought. Although they responded well to soothing in session, they had difficulty self-soothing or soothing each other. They rarely did the homework, but seemed to improve anyway. He was ready to stop therapy. However, she kept bringing up problems and criticisms and he complained that he was always "the bad guy." I (Jen) was feeling cautiously optimistic about their chances.

Things suddenly went nuclear. This week, he had gambled thousands of dollars away and hid that expense from her. After that, he was unlikely to live unbothered in peace and her swoon-worthy delusion evaporated.

Trust can be fragile, but it is essential. It is built over time within an ongoing relationship by many trustworthy acts. He had shattered trust. Therapy was going to take longer than either they or I had believed.

Understanding Trust and Betrayal

How trust is built

Trust is built in the small everyday interactions. Partners offer help when they notice the other person needs it. When there's a history of relationship

DOI: 10.4324/9781003009382-32

problems, trust can be built with consistent refusal to engage in the problem behavior (like alcohol abuse) despite temptations. Offended parties scan the environment for expected breaches in trust and often find them, but at the expense of noticing times of trustworthiness. A forgiveness intervention, or some similar repair, is usually needed to unlock the offended party from knee-jerk lack of trust.

Practiced interactional cycles can build or bust trust

A cycle inspired by the Conflict–Restoration model (Sells et al., 2009) helps couples map their circular conflict cycles involving pain–defense–provocation–pain that erode relational trust (see Figure 26-1). It can be helpful for couples to move from a mysterious, overwhelming flood of emotions to understand their specific cycle and to understand it as a general process all couples face. Few couples can recognize and stop the cycle immediately. So, expecting that is unrealistic. However, using Intervention 26-1 can help couples as they work to repair damage from unproductive conflict. This model is intentionally circular, so there's less blame, which partners will want to do. Partners feel pain, act defensively, and thus provoke the partner and cause the partner pain. The partner reacts defensively, and the cycle of pain–defense–provocation–defense continues. In Intervention 26-1, we discuss how to break free of the cycle.

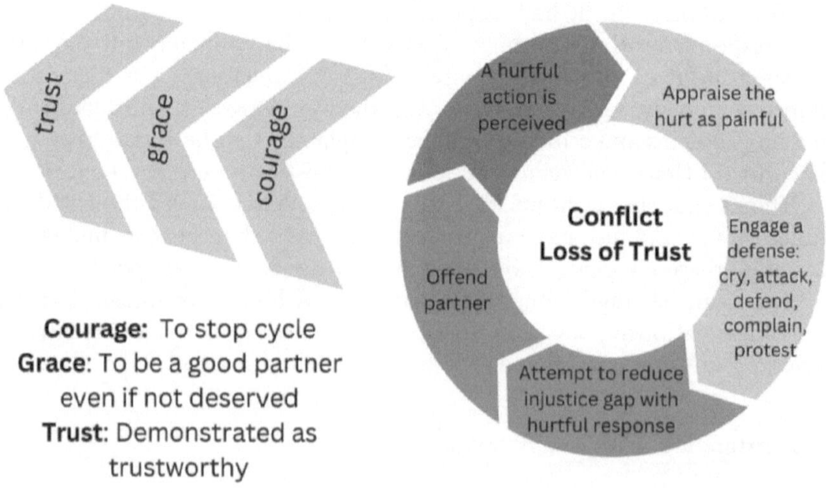

Figure 26-1 Trust

Source: Sells et al., 2009.

Intervention 26-1 Illuminate the Processes of Trust-Busting and Trust-Building

Illuminate trust-busting. After observing a potential pattern, you begin by naming behaviors (i.e., you got hurt, you then felt pain, you got defensive and provoked and hurt your partner, who got defensive and hurt you back). After another repetition or two, you can tentatively speculate that this *might* be a cycle. After another repetition, you can call it definitely a cycle. Once you have the cycle corralled, you can begin to help partners break out.

To stop the cycle will take courage and insight. Here's how it usually happens.

- At least one partner recognizes the cycle as partners are in it.
- The partner interrupts the usual cycle, perhaps saying, "Not today, cycle!"
- Eventually, we would love to get a visceral response like "F#!@ the cycle", in which partners are angry at being trapped in the cycle instead of angry at the partner.
- Partners then have to take a risk. It might be offering a warm hug, a nurturing statement, a time-out, or finding something to agree with the partner.
- One trustworthy instance will not kill the cycle. Trustworthy behaviors must be consistent.

Deep hurts

What if there is a deeply damaging hurt like infidelities, violence, financial bankruptcy, or severe acts of deception? Slow-building trust is the way out (see Intervention 26-2). Rebuilding trust will take a long time and intentional efforts. Partners can expect three steps forward and one or more steps back as they build trust.

Intervention 26-2 Use Slow-Building Trust to Deal with Deep Hurts

The focus of treatment should be on stabilization and immediate needs.

Through your processing with the couple, answer important questions. Should one partner move out for a while to rebuild calm between partners? How will they co-parent? What happens with finances? Can an offending partner tolerate restraints (i.e., an unfaithful partner not seeing the source of the affair; the financially offending partner giving up their credit cards)?

Be alert to and, if you suspect it, assess for psychopathology, disordered personality, and vulnerability of the offender and offended in this situation. Sometimes, pathology feeds the offense cycle. If chronic problems are present, more intensive therapeutic intervention and change will be needed and the couple contract might need renegotiation.

It is vital that couples understand that trust is slow to build up. Now we turn to betrayal of trust. People betray trust for many reasons. Sometimes, opportunities occur. But usually, when people act on those opportunities, they have internal issues that make them open to betraying a trust. Even with extenuating circumstances, most people treat those who betray a trust as responsible—at least to some degree.

Internal factors in betrayal

People don't rationally compute whether to betray a trust. They act implicitly and emotionally in response to opportunities. What makes them open to betraying a trust is usually an implicit "computation" weighing their relationship satisfaction against satisfaction with alternatives and considering the investments in the relationship (i.e., joint friends, shared memories, property owned together, children, etc.; Rusbult et al., 1998).

External factors in betrayal

Besides those implicit "computations," the situation can exert a powerful pull toward betrayal. When we are in a situation, it demands our attention, and situations guide our behavior in many ways we don't fully appreciate. Betrayals can be driven by powerful situations that force people to ignore their implicit "computations" of satisfaction and commitment. Sexual betrayals often happen just because people are near to an available and willing sexual or emotional partner. An offered promotion has seduced many people to abandon their relationship in favor of their job. The desire to be seen as an "insider" in a social situation has seduced many to betray secrets.

Helping Couples Handle a Betrayal of Trust Productively

We can see that responsibility for betrayals of trust is complicated, involving internal and situational pressures, and yet society generally holds people morally culpable when they betray someone. That paradox places couple therapists in tension in conjoint couple therapy. Betrayed partners want us to support them and condemn infidelities—sexual and otherwise. Betrayers don't want to feel judged and might leave therapy if the therapist does not seem supportive. We must craft treatments that walk this tightrope.

So, we now turn to ways that couple therapists can help people handle betrayals of trust well. Such betrayals are among the most difficult ever to forgive. So, it is important to begin by recalling that couples see betrayals as diagnostic moments for the relationship. Trust is built from small moments of turning toward each other, especially when in need. When betrayals occur, those are strong diagnostic moments. Partners highly value the partner's responses in such diagnostic moments because they provide grist for generalizing about the amount one's partner cares for the relationship and oneself as romantic partner.

Help partners process and handle the specific betrayal

When betrayals happen, couple therapists must respond to the betrayal on its own merits. Most couples do not want a glib acrostic, or what feels like a "program," when processing the meaning of emotional betrayals. They need to discuss the specific betrayal. So, the therapist will work with partners to iron out the wrinkles that the betrayal introduced.

After processing, use an acronym to solidify what was learned

After the betrayal has been thoroughly processed, use an acronym to sum up the learning. By understanding the acronym ATTUNE ahead of employing it in session, couple therapists can use its principles to coach partners about how to handle betrayals (Gottman, 2011). Then, after the emotion-laden discussion about the betrayal, the therapist can use the acronym to solidify the principles that emerged (seemingly spontaneously) from processing the betrayal (see Intervention 26-3).

Intervention 26-3 ATTUNE, an Acronym for Handling a Betrayal

After processing betrayals with the couple, couple therapists can help people recall some of the points that probably emerged in the processing. They can use the ATTUNE acronym developed by Gottman (2011).

Attend. Pay attention to what your partner has to say.
Turn toward. Don't turn away from your partner.
Tolerate. Realize that partners have different viewpoints. Tolerating the other's perspective is not the same as agreeing with it.
Understand. Seek to understand internal and external pressures on your partner.
Non-defensive responding. Rather than jumping to defensive responding, respond in a way that keeps communication lines open.
Empathy. Seek to feel with the other; don't get swept up in hurt caused by betrayal.

Help couples anticipate that hurts could happen again

Couples should expect that there will be offenses and possibly perceived betrayals in the future. There could be a re-offense or even less offensive acts that are not intended as betrayals, but might be interpreted that way.

Intervention 26-4 It's Happening Again

A therapist can first collaborate with the couple on identifying offenses related to or similar to the betrayal—for example, an unkind word, a raised voice, or aggression toward an object. If managing anger has been a long-standing struggle for a partner, then understanding that struggle from both partners' perspectives will help.

Therapists can firmly state that the inappropriate behavior is genuinely inappropriate and unacceptable in a loving relationship. And at the same time, expecting never to have any reinjury again is unrealistic.

At this point, many offended partners want to protest. Their #1 goal is NEVER to be hurt like that again. The therapist must help the offended partner differentiate minor offenses from a repeated major injury. If even minor offenses, like a raised voice, are defined as a major injury, then the partner may believe that the relationship will inevitably fail. The partner may be signaling to the therapist that they don't feel safe enough to continue with couple therapy. Another problem in examining potential futures is the fantasy that the relationship will never have problems again.

The therapist should help partners plan for when different levels of reinjury might occur. Responses might be a time-out, cool-down period, or recess until they can discuss the topic in therapy.

Homework questions to help build trust

If partners are building trust, they likely need some activities and exercises that help them (see Intervention 26-5). These are questions partners can answer as homework and bring to therapy. The questions assume both partners have engaged in a breach of trust, which would need adjustment if you had the rare case of a one-way offense.

Intervention 26-5 Partner Exercise in Building Trust

1 What activities are we doing to show we are trustworthy? Are there small, trustworthy things I am trying to do and notice my partner doing?
2 Has there been a good apology? Has the offender shared their understanding of the effects of the loss of trust?
3 Outside of this relationship, how experienced am I at trusting others after a hurt? Is this new and difficult for me? What experiences affect my ability to trust in general?
4 Am I using "I statements" to communicate my need?
5 Are we staying focused on one topic at a time?
6 Can we state aloud our commitment to build trust?
7 Are we willing to share our secrets?

Using a trust bank

Trust is composed of a sense of safety, security, and the ability to rely on the partner in particular areas and in general. Trust requires the trustworthiness of the partner. Trust is like a bank account that can be built or decreased over time. It is vulnerable to a sudden massive "withdrawal" (e.g., a violation of trust) and also hidden charges keep reducing the bank balance (e.g., the wear and tear of daily stresses, strains, and little aggravations that are almost unavoidable). So, it is necessary to continue to add positive actions that convey safety, security, and reliability day by day. Examples of deposits are keeping one's word, keeping the vows sacred and inviolable, doing what is good for the marriage and the partner, and being responsive to bids for attention, sex, or closeness. A particularly important deposit is sacrificing one's self-interest for the partner. Examples of withdrawals that reduce the size of the trust-bank account include lying, failure to follow through on commitments, and not valuing or actively devaluing the partner. Also, it takes many deposits to offset the damage of a small withdrawal. Partners want to keep a positive trust-bank balance.

In Intervention 26-6, we want the partners merely to keep track of trustworthy behaviors, not be on the lookout for the partner's failures in trust. We want them to have an implicit commitment to avoiding betrayals.

Intervention 26-6 The Trust Bank

1 Tell the partners the concept of the Love Bank (Harley, 2022).
2 Explain that the trust bank is different by just tracking trust-building.
3 Suggest that the partners can be an investment adviser for each other, monitoring the partner's behavior for trustworthiness and, when examples are observed, calling attention to them. Suggest that it would not be helpful to point out times when the partner failed to be trustworthy.
4 Describe examples of trustworthiness. These are times when the partner does what they say is intended or what they are responsible for. Give one example, then get each partner to list some things they are responsible for. Do not list things the partner is responsible for.
5 While the exercise is not designed to note failures in trustworthiness, there are times when responsibilities are shirked. Bring up a hypothetical illustration of a failure to be trustworthy For instance, one partner is supposed to shop on Wednesday and fails to do it. Ask the partners what a good response might be. Generally, what you hope they come up with is to trust the partner to do the shopping soon (perhaps the next day) and, therefore, not make a big thing out of it. Portray a partner's failure of trustworthiness as the other partner's opportunity to practice showing trust.

Responding to small failures in trust

Trust is not granted. It is the product of both partners being trustworthy. There are big violations of trust—like affairs. But there are also little violations of trust (e.g., one partner asks the other to do something, and the other fails to carry through). Repeated failures can cause a crisis in trust.

Correct failures quickly. Don't let them build up. Don't let them repeat. This, in many ways, is like a sore finger. If your finger is sore, it seems that you whack it constantly, and you stay aware of it. True, you could die from an infection.

Partners have destroyed many good relationships by getting emotionally focused on one small failure and seeing it as indicative of the entire relationship. In fact, it is a small and abnormal part of an otherwise strong relationship.

Conclusion

Trust is fragile and easily lost in relationships beset by conflict and relational difficulties. If partners have years of faithful interaction with each other, trust has a solid foundation. In troubled relationships, there is little platform of trustworthy behavior to form trust. Partners tend to be suspicious and, in misunderstandings, rarely give the partner the benefit of the doubt. Ruptures occur easily in relationships low in trust. In this chapter, we discussed how to understand trust-building and trust-busting, and we provided interventions to build trust. In the next chapter, we will examine ruptures to the couple's emotional bond and the ways that can be connected to ruptures in the working alliance.

References

Gottman, J. M. (2011). *The Science of Trust: Emotional Attunement for Couples* (First edition.). W. W. Norton.

Harley, W. (2022). *His Needs her Needs: Making Romantic Love Last. Revised and updated.* Revell.

Rusbult, C. E., Martz, J. M., & Agnew, C. R. (1998). The Investment Model Scale: Measuring commitment level, satisfaction level, quality of alternatives, and investment size. *Personal Relationships*, *5*(4), 357–387. https://doi.org/10.1111/j.1475-6811.1998.tb00177.x

Sells, J. N., Beckenbach, J., & Patrick, S. (2009). Pain and defense versus grace and justice: The relational conflict and restoration model. *The Family Journal*, *17*(3), 203–212. https://doi.org/10.1177/1066480709337802

27 Preparing for Future Ruptures

Alert Partners to Inevitable Future Ruptures

Problem:	Relationships will not be perfect after therapy ends.
Solution:	Prepare couples to address future ruptures with improved relationship care.

We studied over 150 early-married couples (Worthington et al., 2015) who received nine hours of individual couple enrichment. We followed them for five assessment periods from pre-treatment to over a year post-treatment. The couples were recruited at six months post-marriage, so by the end of the study, they had been married from 18 to 24 months. The counselors were professional post-degree licensed counselors, social workers, or psychologists. We compared the "handling our problems effectively" (HOPE) half of the hope-focused couple approach (HFCA) (consisting of assessment, feedback, resolution of differences, communication, and intimacy) against the "forgiveness and reconciliation through experiencing intimacy" (FREE) half of the approach, and against an assessment-only condition in which people were assessed repeatedly without intervention or feedback. The results surprised us.

The HOPE and FREE interventions had immediate and lasting positive effects on the couples. That didn't surprise us. Those in HOPE had slightly better results on couple satisfaction at the end of treatment, but those effects decayed to about half what they were by the follow-up period. They were still positive but less positive than for those in FREE. However, those couples in the FREE intervention had immediate and substantial gains, and those gains did not decay by the follow-up. Couples in the assessment-only condition were progressively less satisfied with their relationship, consistent with much research on untreated early-married couples in their first couple of years of marriage.

DOI: 10.4324/9781003009382-33

We were careful to tell all couples that these treatments would not prevent problems in their marriage but should help them cope with the problems when they arose. The results suggested to us that not all of the couples believed us.

Despite our framing HOPE as a coping treatment, couples trained in HOPE often believed that the meta-message of communication-conflict their training was that they should not have future problems because they now knew how to communicate. So, by the end of the counseling, they had strong gains in satisfaction. But, when inevitable difficulties arose, they lost half of their gains.

On the other hand, the meta-message of FREE training was that they would have problems that required forgiveness and reconciliation. So, they benefited by forgiving hurts during treatment but when later problems arose after treatment, their forgiveness and reconciliation skills helped maintain their gains.

What We Learned from Our Research

Our lesson was clear. In spite of how we frame our treatments, prepare couples for potential ruptures in the emotional bond to the extent we can. To prepare couples, we must predict potential ruptures. There will be several ways we can anticipate them. The primary method is to engage in ongoing weekly assessment—routine outcome monitoring. That way, we see storm clouds gathering. Second, be alert to resistance and roadblocks. Third, recognize that difficult individual problems, like trauma or personality disorders, will often spell trouble for couples. Fourth, listen to your reactions to partners. They sometimes tell you that your bonds with them are weak, which can also alert you to be vigilant about potential ruptures the couple. If their confidence in you is collapsing, you might anticipate that this will show up with them.

Once you have become alert to potential ruptures in the couple's emotional bond, try to forestall it by talking about the potential danger, shifting course if needed, and thinking ahead about what you might do if the rupture in emotional closeness manifests.

Anticipating Ruptures in Emotional Closeness

Therapists are not very good at knowing from therapy how well couples are doing. Generally, clinicians rate their clients as experiencing more positive change than (a) clients rate themselves, (b) objective measures reveal, or (c) impartial observers estimate. This is not surprising. We are, after all, really invested in the couple's success. We also have limited data to work with. We see the couple only in session. In a session, we are front and center for them. That, to some degree, controls their negative behaviors. So, this should give us pause at relying on our impressions of the couples.

Assess throughout therapy

We need to ask partners to assess their relationships directly. We have identified several areas you might assess using questions in therapy or finding established measures —working alliance, emotional bond, hope, work, love, and progress toward goals. Interventions that focus on observing change throughout therapy (such as those described below with 27-1, 27-2, 27-3 and 27-4) will help prepare for ruptures that are inevitable throughout treatment.

Intervention 27-1 Anticipate Ruptures by Assessing Change throughout Treatment

Routine Outcome Monitoring (ROM). We can anticipate some ruptures by asking partners to complete a quick assessment (about three minutes) at the outset of each session while waiting for the session to begin. We ask directly about six areas we identified as important using the Hope weekly couple's assessment (see Chapter 11).

The purpose of periodic assessment is to induce clinical change or prevent clinical deterioration. ROM can increase motivation and prompt re-evaluating progress toward goals. The discussion in response to the assessment can help partners mark progress.

We treat couple therapy as a collaborative, patient-centered approach. If you give clients an active role in their therapy, they will improve more in objective outcomes (Owen et al., 2012). Think of your own experience. All medical appointments you attend require time-demanding online self-reports of your status before every appointment. Then, just to be sure, the nurse reviews the same questions in person. Clients also are used to this. We need not hesitate to ask our couples to complete three minutes of questions each week.

Stay calm when you meet resistances or roadblocks

We distinguish between a resistance and a roadblock. *Resistance* is an inner psychological barrier to change. In contrast, a *roadblock* is something external that impedes counseling. It may be business, financial strain, illness, or other situational impediment.

Intervention 27-2 Anticipate Ruptures by Staying Calm in the Face of Resistances and Roadblocks

Try not to get hung up on whether the barrier is internal or external. They are often intertwined.

Instead, seek to understand the barrier to progress. Work with the couple to determine how to knock down, climb over, go around, or tunnel beneath the barrier. For a time, getting past the barrier can become a short-term intermediate goal, and hopefully they will be past it within a few sessions.

Importantly, resistances and roadblocks can frustrate both you and the couple. So, stay warm and supportive. If you deal calmly with resistance and roadblocks, you can often avoid frustrations that lead to ruptures in emotional closeness and ruptures in your working alliance with the partners.

Be especially alert when a partner has a history of trauma

Trauma histories, regardless of whether a partner meets the criteria for post-traumatic stress disorder (PTSD), are fraught. Triggers often populate relationships like landmines. So, when you encounter couples in which one partner (or both) has a trauma history, look for triggers that might rupture the emotional bond between partners or damage the working alliance with you.

Intervention 27-3 Anticipate Ruptures When Working with Partners Who Have a Trauma History

Step 1: Assess trauma history. To anticipate potential ruptures, give special attention to the traumatic event and how the person copes with it. This might involve assessing the trauma history and functioning—not as detailed as treating the person for PTSD, but rather assessing the likelihood of a flare-up interfering with couple therapy. According to one of the most respected researchers in the field, George Bonanno (2021), only about 15 percent of potentially traumatic events produce diagnosable traumas for people experiencing them. Most people are resilient. They bounce back within a few weeks. Or they recover more slowly but do not have lasting post-traumatic symptoms.

Step 2: Address trauma history. When both partners know the trauma history and when it is interfering with the relationship, address it. There are resources for clinicians working with couples with PTSD (Monson & Fredman, 2012; Wagner et al., 2016).

Step 3: Identify triggers. After you've assessed the extent of the impairment due to the trauma, help the couple identify triggers within their relationship. This often requires sensitivity by therapists because identifying triggers can become a trigger itself to re-experiencing the remembered traumatic situation and emotional experience.

Step 4: Watch your step. The general guideline is to be slow and careful. Walking through a minefield is a metaphor that resonates with therapists dealing with an easily triggered PTSD client. The analogy seems apt in many cases of couple therapy. Slow and careful approach helps the partner who experiences triggers to calm themselves and not be catapulted into emotional flooding. It also aids the partner in understanding the triggers and finding more effective responses to them.

Be sensitive to your own reactions to partners

Our emotional reactions to one or both partners are sometimes our best diagnostic devices. Ev still remembers now, almost 45 years later, counseling a pastor and his spouse. They had been to three previous couple therapists. They were unsatisfied with each. At the first assessment session, the pastor gave Ev a "theological examination" within five minutes of the greeting. Duh. That should have been a cue.

After three couple therapy sessions, it was clear that therapy was not helpful. Almost every session turned into a critique of Ev's flawed theology, some unhelpful intervention, or banal homework. During the fourth session, we had a hard conversation about ending therapy. I made a referral to another therapist in town. The pastor expressed disappointment in Ev, in therapy as being consistent with the pastor's theology, and in his marriage.

Ev's reactions to the husband were strong and negative. Starting about six minutes deep into their first meeting. That should have been an immediate message that conveyed danger to the working alliance and (by projecting onto the wife) the emotional bond. How could any emotional bond stand the daily onslaught of criticism and judgment, not only as a person but as a Christian!? Yet, in his inexperience, Ev did not listen to his feelings and wasted the time and money of the couple and his own time (and self-esteem).

At a holiday party in Richmond, Ev saw the seasoned therapist to whom he had referred the couple. Ev asked whether the therapist had treated the couple. "I fired them from therapy before the first session ended," he said. "I could tell by my own reaction that that relationship was probably headed for divorce. I found later that they had tried couple therapy with at least seven total therapists, and none could help. I don't know what they did after that last therapist. I wouldn't be surprised if they divorced."

Intervention 27-4 Anticipate Ruptures by Monitoring the Therapist's Own Negative Reactions

A client's interpersonal stance will "pull" for the couple therapist to feel and behave in certain ways. So, how we feel compelled to respond to a partner can give us clues about what their partner might be feeling. Or not. Clinical judgment is required.

Make time to reflect on your feelings. Jen has found it helpful to sit down at the end of the intake or assessment session and reflect on her feelings about each partner. She often finds interpersonal patterns have already developed. When a partner is complimentary and defers easily, that pulls for her to act like an expert or parent—not the best stance to take in collaborative, patient-centered couple therapy. Also, she thinks about whether that same deference was shown with the partner, which could be informative about their relationship. Similarly, if a client withholds information and friendly expression, that sometimes can trigger suspicion or might make us want to try hard to please the person. That might indicate that partners might have trust issues, and the other partner might either be a doormat or might have dismissed the withholder saying, "I don't care what he thinks."

You will use clinical judgment about how to use your personal reactions. For some therapists, that is important grist for the therapy mill. For others, they avoid referring to it unless therapy sputters. Then, using personal reactions might kick it into gear again.

Conclusion

When Jen supervises clinicians in her training clinic, most of the attention in supervision focuses on ruptures in the couple bond or therapist–couple alliance. The wide variety of indicators of rupture is a never-ending source of amazement. People are creative at resistance and roadblocks. The therapist who can maintain compassion, care, and connection while firmly communicating an expectation of work and progress has the best chance to work through roadblocks and ruptures.

A saying in our clinic is, "This is why they pay us the big bucks; otherwise, they could just read things off the internet and get better." This work is challenging but deeply rewarding for couples who can work courageously through their blocks.

References

Bonanno, G. A. (2021). *The End of Trauma: How the New Science of Resilience is Changing How We Think About PTSD*. Basic Books.

Monson, C. M. & Fredman, S. J., (2012). *Cognitive-Behavioral Conjoint Therapy for PTSD: Harnessing the Healing Power of Relationships*. New York: Guilford Press.

Owen, J., Anker, M., Duncan, B., & Sparks, J. (2012). Initial relationship goal and couple therapy outcomes at post and six-month follow-up. *Journal of Family Psychology*, 26(2), 179–186. https://doi.org/10.1037/a0026998

Wagner, A. C., Monson, C. M., & Hart, T. L. (2016). Understanding social factors in the context of trauma: Implications for measurement and intervention. *Journal of Aggression, Maltreatment, & Trauma, 25*, 831–853.

Worthington, E. L., Jr., Berry, J. W., Hook, J. N., Davis, D. E., Scherer, M., Griffin, B. J., Wade, N. G., Yarhouse, M., Ripley, J. S., Miller, A. J., Sharp, C. B, Canter, D. E., & Campana, K. L. (2015). Forgiveness–reconciliation and communication-conflict-resolution interventions versus rested controls in early married couples. *Journal of Counseling Psychology*, 62(1), 14–27.

28 Solidifying Gains at Termination

Promote Reflective Future Planning in Light of Review of Therapy

Problem:	The gains of couple therapy can be easily lost after couple therapy.
Solution:	Use intentional strong interventions and follow-up plans at the end of treatment to solidify gains.

We have found it humbling to talk to couples who went through the hope-focused couple approach (HFCA). When they are successful, we ask what they found to be the most helpful in couple therapy. Typically, they say they achieved their goals (i.e., "We restored our love"), found therapy positive ("We found it challenging at times, but a good experience" or "We got to talk things out without too much arguing"), or were positively affected by their therapist ("We learned a lot from your wisdom"—aw, shucks, thanks).

Few couples have said, "Wow, I really enjoyed intervention 14-3." The techniques to help partners change, that we therapists spend so much time thinking about, don't bubble to the top of partners' memory. Partners don't remember everything that happened in therapy or why it helped them improve their relationship. We aren't blaming couples for not attributing their successes to what we did. In fact, if they did, we have failed to use a patient-centered approach. Instead, they see things from their perspective, focusing on what they put time and effort into, not what we put time and effort into. And this is a good thing. We want them to attribute their success to personal, global, positive, and stable factors. Their courageous effort. Their willingness to risk new things. Their ability to learn.

Not all of the couples we talk to have successful experiences. We still learn important things from them. Early dropout in couple therapy is often understood as a mismatch of what the couple wants compared to what couple therapy offers. This is not always true. Some issues might simply

DOI: 10.4324/9781003009382-34

not be addressable by therapy. These could include severe financial pressures, making couple therapy less important than paying overdue bills. Also, a health crisis (like psychotic event or stroke) makes couple therapy less important than survival. For others, time constraints, such as elder care, could make finding time for couple therapy difficult. But couples do terminate prematurely for several other reasons.

1 Some couples have already taken steps to end the relationship and they follow through.
2 Others can't alter unrealistic expectations that a therapist will take their side and correct their spouse.
3 Some couples stick with counseling for a while but conclude they are not making the progress they hoped for. This might be because they held overly optimistic expectations of quick success. Or because they had a crisis and became dejected. Or because they believed they were better off than the average couple so additional sessions would not help much.

If you've assessed routinely, we hope you will not be caught off guard by an early termination or simply a permanent no-show, because you saw it coming through assessment results. Using routing outcome monitoring (ROM) to identify when progress is poor, you might derail premature termination tendencies before the couple considers it. You might help couples discuss their roadblocks or resistances before they crash. By looking at a couple's ROM data, you can observe that you noticed that their scores have not changed much (or have gotten worse) and ask what's going on. You could ask whether they believe couple therapy should be refocused. You could ask whether they want to change their treatment plan. If you've routinely assessed, any of those might be possible.

But what if therapy ends well. What is the essence of a good termination? That is where we want to spend the bulk of the time in this chapter.

Tasks of Termination

There are three general tasks to accomplish in a successful termination.

1 Review how to make change last. This involves reviewing what worked and what didn't work and identifying things the couple could do to maintain gains.
2 Create a memorable bonding event between the partners.
3 Have a meaningful goodbye that signifies a celebration of what was accomplished but a transition to independence from the couple therapist.

These three things need to be "sticky." They need to stick to the couple as they leave couple therapy so the gains in couple therapy last. Let's look closer at these tasks.

What worked and what still needs work?

Much of the discussion during termination should identify which aspects of counseling affected the couple the most. If you limit those to three important experiences, the partners will most likely remember them. More is not better.

Successful couples often want to acknowledge the contributions of the therapist. We certainly appreciate that when it happens (and we should tell them so), but that won't help them maintain gains. However, general positive feelings about the therapist might make it more likely that they seek couple therapy if problems recur or new ones develop.

Intervention 28-1 Three Questions at Termination

Focus on what the partners did and what the couple did together. Ask,

1 "What did you do together that most helped make your relationship better?"
2 "What did your partner do that helped your relationship improve?"
3 "How do you think you have grown as a person during this couple therapy?"

These three questions can be good journaling homework for the couple before the termination sessions.

Some couple therapists might take notes during termination discussions and give a photocopy to each partner at the end of the session while adding the original to their case notes. One clear message should be, "You worked hard and improved your relationship during therapy. One lesson from that is that you could do this again if you ever needed to." This increases their sense of efficacy in repairing their relationship, hope, and motivation to deal positively with adverse reactions if (when) they occur in the future.

In every couple therapy, some areas were not attended to or not long enough. You'll find out the most about what worked and what still needs work because you do a final assessment (in the next to last session) and then provide written feedback that you discuss with the partners. Couples take the same measures they took at the intake.

The therapist compares the original and final assessment results and organizes them into a report. That is typically not quite as easy as the initial assessment, which tends to follow a template. The therapist can copy from the initial report, saving time. The final report can also be targeted to the primary goals of therapy and reflecting on them, rather than educating the couple about couple therapy as the intake report does.

The comparison is a powerful intervention for many couples. For couples where both partners have improved, there is confirmation that their relationship has improved. Using charts or graphs helps the couple visualize changes in the relationship in different areas of functioning. Any charts or graphs must be tailored to the education level of the couple. It is better to use simple, easily understood graphics than to give every detail of assessment (see Figure 28-1).

We often give average scores on a scale or measure instead of the total score, which is more readily understood by the partners and easy to graph, either by hand or with a computer program.

While you'll want to have a narrative discussion about changes that have happened during therapy, sometimes showing couples the quantitative graph of the changes in the scores over time makes a big impact quickly. At the final assessment, encourage couples who need further growth in their relationship with specific written suggestions. In times of difficulty, the chances they will re-read the final report are much greater than that they will remember verbal communication.

The final termination report can help make treatment more memorable and review what happened in therapy. (We have provided an abbreviated example of one in Intervention 28-2.) It summarizes the actual treatment plan, which might differ from the one initially proposed. That helps review the flow of therapy. It evaluates the progress of reaching therapy goals, by comparing assessment results in the penultimate session with initial results. It suggests potential goals for the partners to work on and sets a tentative date for a post-treatment follow-up check-up. You can keep the words brief in the report, and use your discussion to encourage and elaborate as needed.

Intervention 28-2 An Example of a Final Termination Report

David and Danielle

We had 15 sessions of therapy across six months. Your original goal was to decrease conflict related to Danielle's panic attacks, increase co-parenting cooperation, and better understand your relationship.

Week-by-Week Results

If you used weekly measures for satisfaction, conflict, communication, intimacy, etc., you could include a weekly data presentation here perhaps graphically.

Pre-Post Couple Satisfaction Measure

David pre-counseling: 3.4 (somewhat dissatisfied) and end-counseling 5.1 (usually satisfied).

Danielle pre-counseling: 3.1 (somewhat dissatisfied) and end-counseling 4.6 (usually satisfied).

See graph (Figure 28-1).

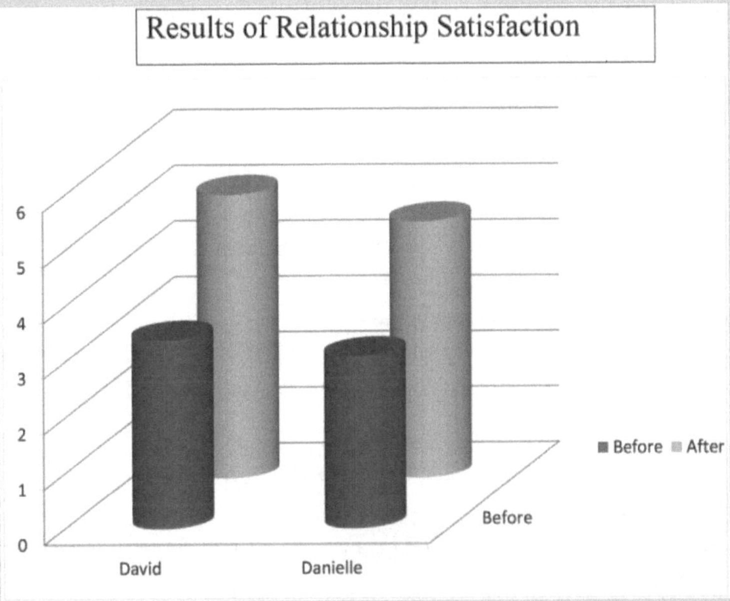

Figure 28-1 Figure in Termination Report Reporting the Results of Relationship Closeness Before Therapy (darker pillars) and After Therapy (lighter pillars)

Pre-Post Couple Efficacy Measure (Ability to solve problems you face)

David pre-counseling: 3.4 (lower efficacy) and end-counseling 6.1 (good efficacy).

Danielle pre-counseling: 3.1 (lower efficacy) and end-counseling 5.5 (somewhat good efficacy).

Graphs could be used on each pre-post report.

Pre-Post Couple Trust Measure

David pre-counseling: 4.4 (usually trusting) and end-counseling 5.1 (trusting).
Danielle pre-counseling: 4.8 (trusting) and end-counseling 5.4 (trusting).

Narrative Summary and Recommendations

You can see from the objective data that you have each improved on individual measures and together, looking at preliminary report and the current data, you can see that you've improved. As we finish, I have three major recommendations.

1 Maintain good boundaries around your family, especially when your work and extended family attempt to intrude.
2 The conversations in which you listened to each other's needs inspired me. I encourage you to keep finding good times to talk about your needs with each other. Several times a month, ask your spouse, "What needs should I be aware of in your life this week?"
3 Your ability to have time together, just the two of you, is especially difficult right now. Make an appointment with yourselves to talk about how you can find some positive "date night" time together in your current phase of life.

It would be helpful to consider a six-month check-up either by phone (gratis) or another round of assessments (paid) if you suspect that more therapy would be helpful.

I enjoyed working with you as you have courageously improved your marriage.
/Signed/

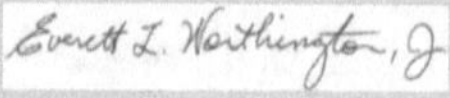

Final Emotional Bonding Event

As couple therapy ends, it is important to create a memorable event that turns them even more toward each other and makes final improvements on their attachment. One intervention commonly used near the end of the HFCA is Intervention 28-3 called either the Joshua Memorial or graduation ceremony, depending on the beliefs of the partners. If both partners are practicing their faith or are open to the stories of the Abrahamic faiths, we generally use "Joshua Memorial." The name came from the Hebrew Scriptures (Joshua 4:1-7). When Joshua led the Israelites into the promised land, he established a monument by taking 12 stones from the Jordan River—one selected by a representative of each of the 12 tribes. With our secular clients or people who embrace a different (non-Abrahamic) religion, we rename this their graduation ceremony. This depends on our clinical judgment about their spiritual values.

Intervention 28-3 Joshua Memorial or Graduation Ceremony

In the session before the termination session, the couple is told that a task most couples have benefited from is designing a symbol of their progress during therapy. This will be a memorial intended to be displayed in their home to remind them of their accomplishments in therapy.

Give some examples. These include couples who have written and recorded a song about treatment. One couple encased the LOVE acronym in plastic and framed it for display. Another couple had a weekend away on week 16, and they framed a picture at the lodge they stayed at.

In the final session, the couple brings their memorial. They talk about why they benefited from therapy and what they want to remember from it.

We like this intervention because creating their memorial requires partners to think through what was meaningful in couple therapy and translate it into something that makes change sensible to them. It thus is patient-centered and it reinforces their autonomy, which is important at their launch from treatment. It also helps promote the emotional bond between partners because they work on this together and develop a non-rational symbol of their progress.

The intervention can go awry. Try to anticipate possible troubles in advance. On the few times when it has blown up, one partner has had little involvement in the creation, citing "I'm not creative." If only one partner creates the memorial, there is no sense of shared meaning. Also, the partner who did most of the work can interpret the other partner's lack of participation as a lack of engagement in the relationship. Diffuse the "I'm not creative" defense ahead of time. Say, when assigning it, that the assignment is not an exercise in mere creativity. Both partners can contribute by providing ideas and lending a hand in whatever work was done to make the memorial. The counselor can help avoid a one-sided memorial by encouraging the couple to understand the importance of the work of creation together.

Checking Up Post-Therapy

One challenging aspect of couples therapy is the high recidivism rate. Couples can return to old habits and dysfunctional patterns once their energy and attention have shifted away from couple therapy. This is especially true if they terminate before the completion of the (final) rehabilitation phase of couple therapy. Some research has studied long-term effects of couple therapy (Owen et al., 2012). Results are disappointing for one-, two-, and five-year outcomes. Because long-term effects are not uniformly good, following up at six months post-therapy is a good idea.

Intervention 28-4 Post-Therapy Assessment

Some therapists use these check-ups for brief assessments. The therapist is one of the beneficiaries of a follow-up session with a couple. Several months after therapy has ended, the couple can communicate what has been retained, which helps therapists see what interventions were powerful.

We have found that the most effective way to ensure that a post-therapy follow-up becomes a regular part of your practice is to include it in pre-therapy information, discuss it during the intake period as a regular part of practice, and build in the cost so that the cost of the six-month "check-up" has been paid as part of the normal course of therapy.

Conclusion

Most couple therapy does not end with intentional, intense interventions like we recommend for HFCA. We believe this is one of the secrets to our long-term efficacy (Ripley et al., 2021). Our research found that 2 to 10 years after treatment couples who completed treatment had maintained gains or continued to improve. While we don't have the research (yet) to substantiate our claim, we find the Joshua Memorial/graduation ceremony, final assessment with feedback, and post-therapy check-up help end couple therapy in a positive, memorable, "sticky" way while taking recidivism of gains seriously.

We now approach the end of our journey through couple therapy. In the final chapter, we summarize just a few of the major lessons we hope you take away from this book.

References

Owen, J., Anker, M., Duncan, B., & Sparks, J. (2012). Initial relationship goal and couple therapy outcomes at post and six-month follow-up. *Journal of Family Psychology*, 26(2), 179–186. https://doi.org/10.1037/a0026998

Ripley, J., Solfelt, L., Ord, A., Garthe, R. C., Worthington, E. L., & Channing, T. (2021). Short- and long-term outcomes of hope-focused couple therapy. *Spirituality in Clinical Practice*. https://doi.org/10.1037/scp0000286

29 Reaching a Productive Conclusion

Heed these Take-Home Messages

Problem:	In a long book on couple therapy, what are the main take-aways?
Solution:	In patient-responsive couple therapy aimed at promoting a stronger emotional bond, use your strategy, know enough techniques to be flexible, and help partners stay hopeful.

In Chapter 7, we identified 13 principles that we thought captured the essence of the hope-focused couple approach (HFCA). These included things like, of first importance, be patient-responsive. In today's consumer climate, that is required. Also, we emphasized being positive, using evidence-based techniques, focusing on hope, using explicit assessment, and developing a patient-responsive treatment plan and sticking to it, regardless of provocation of crises du jour. We have tried to stay relationship-focused rather than technique-focused even though one of the strengths of the book, we hope, is to enhance your repertoire of techniques. Even though we began with these important principles, we knew that we would be unfolding a great story between that beginning and this chapter that details what we believe are important take-home messages. We know that you have come at this book based on your own experience, expectations, values, and beliefs. So, we know that your take-homes might differ from ours. Nevertheless, we wanted to close the book by reflecting on what we believe are important lasting lessons. We actually selected others but we relegated them to supplemental material that can be found at www.hopecouples.com. Here are what we think are the major lessons.

There Is a Logic Involved in Successful Couple Therapy

There is a logic to HFCA treatment. Outcomes are dependent on repairing and rebuilding the *emotional bond*, which is the cause of good

DOI: 10.4324/9781003009382-35

relationships—both between partners and between the couple and couple therapist. The emotional bond between couple and therapist is best enhanced through patient-responsive behavior. We focus on increasing *hope* so that people will work on strengthening their emotional bond. There is an overall *strategy* of promoting love, work, and faith that leads to hope. *Techniques* provide tactical options for achieving the strategy.

Effective couple therapy is patient-responsive, relationship-centered, and collaborative

Despite our emphasis on techniques, we hope the message comes through clearly that we believe the relationship between the couple therapist and each individual partner is the cornerstone of effectiveness. This seems to be an era in which Western couples are rejecting authority-based approaches in favor of collaborative ones. Since the beginning, the HFCA has emphasized responding empathically to couples and partners. Sometimes, that is a difficult balancing act for sure, but we believe that it is vital to keep patient autonomy at the forefront of treatment. By providing timely feedback about what you see as going on and listening to partners, you keep the relationship patient-responsive, relationship-centered, and collaborative.

Effective couple therapy strengthens the emotional bond between partners through strategic intervention

That emotional bond, which is a sense of closeness and connection between the partners that binds them into a "couple" instead of two individuals, is related to each individual's adult attachment. However, the emotional bond is a relational quality. As such, it involves a lot more than an individual's attachment style. By focusing on love as valuing the partner and not devaluing the partner, the approach uses language that is used by and easily understood by couples. Emphasizing the importance of putting energy (i.e., work) into the relationship keeps partners engaged in sessions and after termination. Emphasizing faith in oneself, one's partner, and the effectiveness of therapy keeps partners receptive to building trust.

Couple therapy has three phases, all aimed to bring about more hope

The phases affect the conduct of techniques and provide natural transition points in treatment. Each phase builds upon the previous one. The initial phase is about recapturing hope. It includes assessment and feedback sessions and the first two or three treatment sessions, usually (but not always) on conflict negotiation. The danger of premature termination is great if, after initial gains, a negative relationship event occurs. In the second phase, symptoms of a troubled relationship are addressed and (hopefully) ameliorated. Hope is solidified by the usually gradual, but sometimes sudden, two-step-forward-one-step-back progress. Some research on psychotherapy shows that sudden change in individual psychotherapy is experienced in about 40 percent of the cases (Hayes et al., 2007). In most cases, they never experience a spurt forward in functioning. This 40 percent sudden-change number is good to share with couples during feedback because it helps set expectations. Danger of premature termination is greatest (1) if change is stagnated or (2) just after a spurt forward. In the third phase, the couple tries to return to functioning "normally." This takes time, and some couples might simply tire of couple therapy and desire to terminate early.

Techniques are important, but remember the grand strategy

There are many determinants of the success of therapy. These include things like the personality of the individual partners, the relationship between the partners, and the specifics of the partners' lives. The choices of approach and specific techniques are really the only things under the control of the therapist. So, we need to choose the things we can control wisely.

Assessment of the partners and the relationship is one key to selecting the best technique. Besides matching techniques to problems, we also match techniques to strengths. When learning a new approach to therapy, it is easy to get caught up in the minutia of techniques and try to implement them perfectly. Perfect delivery of technique is not the key to your best work. Keep in mind the grand strategy.

- The emotional bond is the centerpiece of the grand strategy.
- A strategy of faith, work, and love guides you.
- Hope provides energy for change.
- Techniques flow from these.
- Improved outcomes—satisfaction, maturity, and stability—are signs that the grand plan is working.

You need good techniques to help resolve conflicts, improve communication, and increase intimacy. Near the end of therapy, partners will likely need to detoxify the relationship. Forgiveness and reconciliation are great ways of doing so, but don't neglect things like restoring justice, turning the matter over to God, forbearing, and accepting. Building devotion into the relationship is not simple. Although the positive is focused on all along, in addition to solving problems, the last phase of reconciling represents a shift from problem-focus to solution-focus.

Many common problems in couple therapy can be understood and addressed through routine outcome monitoring (ROM). It's important to make this process simple, natural, and routine so that it will happen. But once employed, both the clients and therapist can address roadblocks and resistances, as well as celebrate gains in treatment.

Termination is vital to stamp in a couple's learning and set them on the road to a grand future. This spans the time frame of their relationship. You will want to get them to review the past and get them to come up with a "graduation ritual." Then, you'll want to get them to survey the present functioning of their relationship. And finally, you'll give feedback that helps them plan to keep moving forward into the future.

Hope is realistic

Hope is not pie-in-the-sky optimism. It is grounded in real-life struggle. Just because you embrace the HFCA, or seek to promote hope in whatever approach you use, does not mean you are not aware of difficulties. One of the most difficult parts of couple therapy as a therapist is seeing couples who have a mountain of struggle. Sometimes, couple therapists show up to supervision or seek peer supervision because they are bedraggled, trying so hard to do a good job with a couple overloaded with problems and limited in motivation. It's easy to get discouraged. But what you are doing in couple therapy (and supervision of couple therapists) is a noble work. But it's hard. It takes a massive amount of work to steer a battleship out of a minefield.

Conclusion

In this book, we have tried to provide tools that you can use in your practice of couple therapy. The tools have been mostly techniques, but we've also sought to give you reasons behind the techniques and behind the logic for choosing them. The techniques have almost always been those that relied on more tangible actions than just talking about the relationship. Talk is vital, but so is active involvement with tangible actions or items. We have tried to provide a broad-based meta-theoretical framework that centers on several levels using a grand strategy. Armed with state-of-the-practice tools, your wealth of experience, and a commitment to excellence, you can succeed, and we wish you the best of success in your treatment of couples.

Reference

Hayes, A. M. Laurenceau, J.-P., Feldman, G., Strauss, J. L., & Cardaciotto, L. A. (2007). Change is not always linear: The study of nonlinear and discontinuous patterns of change in psychotherapy. *Clinical Psychology Review, 27*(6), 715–723. https://doi.org/10.1016/j.cpr.2007.01.008

Index

Bold page numbers indicate tables, *italic* numbers indicate figures.